Pelican Books

Phobias

Ross Mitchell studied medicine at Edinburgh University and psychiatry at St Francis Hospital, Haywards Heath. He was a psychiatrist with the R.A.M.C., and at Barrow Guerney Hospital, Bristol. He is currently Consultant Psychiatrist to Fulbourn and Addenbrooke's Hospitals, Cambridge. He is particularly interested in community psychiatry and works directly with general practitioners, nurses and social workers in Health Centres. Dr Mitchell is married with two children. Penguin have also published his book *Depression*.

ROSS MITCHELL

Penguin Books

PHOBIAS

Penguin Books Ltd, Harmondsworth, Middlesex, England
Penguin Books, 625 Madison Avenue, New York, New York 10022, U.S.A.
Penguin Books Australia Ltd, Ringwood, Victoria, Australia
Penguin Books Canada Ltd, 2801 John Street, Markham, Ontario, Canada L3R 1B4
Penguin Books (N.Z.) Ltd, 182–190 Wairau Road, Auckland 10, New Zealand

First published 1982

Photoset in Linotron Univers by Rowland Phototypesetting Ltd, Bury St Edmunds, Suffolk
Made and printed in Great Britain by Hazel, Watson and Viney Ltd, Aylesbury, Buckinghamshire

Contents

To Rhoda, Nicola and Michael

Thus conscience doth make cowards of us all.
SHAKESPEARE

Prosperity is not without many fears and distastes; and adversity is not without comforts and hopes.
BACON

No, when the fight begins within himself,
A man's worth something . . .
BROWNING

Introduction

Anxiety and fear are among the greatest enemies we have to face as human beings: anxiety about our vulnerability, and fear for our very survival. We are threatened from without by wars, famines and all kinds of disasters, but we are also threatened from within by powerful forebodings about our more immediate futures. Faced with uncertainty about what may happen to us, we remain insecure and anxious.

For some the objects of those fears are shared with everyone else, a common inheritance, but for others the same terrors are released by what, in the eyes of most, are trivial causes and not worth bothering about. These others are the sufferers of *phobias*, who go through agonies and untold distress at the thought of having to face quite ordinary experiences – going shopping, travelling on public transport, visiting the cinema, dining out in a restaurant, being in a room with a cat or a dog, even being out on their own in the streets.

People with phobias are faced with two sources of distress – the situation which holds such terrors for them and the knowledge that others do not share the same fears, believing them to be foolish, weak and stupid. 'How can you be afraid of travelling in a bus?' 'Whoever heard of anyone being afraid of the supermarket?' 'You're not really terrified of thunder, are you?' Their misery is compounded as they begin to doubt themselves. Perhaps they *are* weak and stupid; perhaps they *are* going out of their minds. Slowly, as they try to avoid all the sources of their distress, their lives become more and more restricted, until finally they may become virtual prisoners in their own homes, the only place where they can still feel reasonably safe and secure.

How common are such phobias? How do people come to suffer from them? What can be done to help someone with a phobia which traps them in their home, or at least limits severely what they are able to do? What happens in families when one parent is markedly phobic? Can it affect the children? What can the partner do to help?

This book will try to answer these questions and will try to make sense of something which, by its nature, does not seem to make sense. After all, we all get worried from time to time; we all have to face difficult and distressing situations as part of everyday life. Why are some people so upset about such relatively minor things, when there are so many real worries to concern us?

CHAPTER 1
THE NATURE OF ANXIETY

Anxiety, as we all know to our cost, is a highly unpleasant experience which we try to avoid if we can. This unpleasantness is difficult to describe, but we can say that it has two components: what we feel in our minds, in our consciousness of ourselves, and what we observe in our bodies. In our minds there is a heightened awareness of tension and uneasiness, an apprehension of forthcoming distress, which is itself distressing. This makes us restless and drives us to do something either to get rid of the source of the anxiety or to run away from it. In our bodies there is the familiar 'butterflies in the stomach' – a feeling of tension which, if severe enough, makes us think we might be sick. Our hearts beat faster, our hands tremble and sweat more than usual. There is pressure to go to the lavatory which at times is uncontrollable. Others notice that we are pale and look ill-at-ease. If this anxiety gets very much worse, there is an overwhelming sense of dread, the sense of something awful about to happen – either that we shall faint, which we may do, or that our hearts will stop, or that we shall go out of our minds soon if there is no release. In the face of such anxiety, we lose all our composure and feel that whatever self-confidence we may have had is quickly ebbing away. In this way, heroes may fear that they are in danger of being made into cowards.

Such inner, subjective anxiety levels can be measured objectively by assessing the physiological changes in the body – an increase of heart rate and respiration, a rise in blood pressure, a fall of electrical resist-

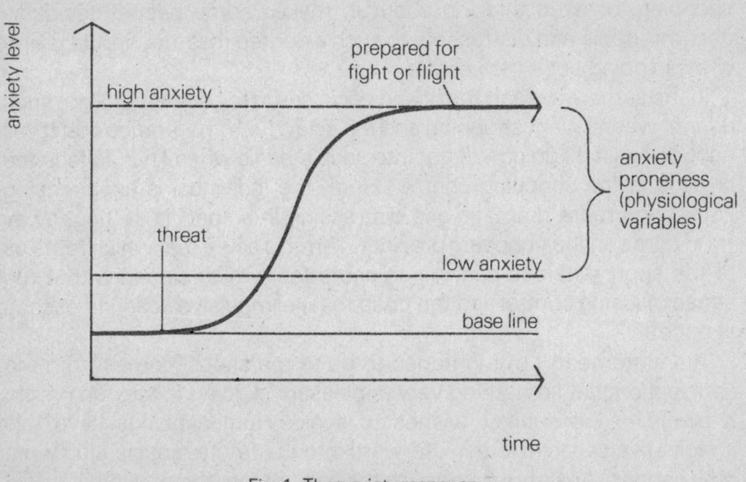

Fig. 1 The anxiety response

ance of the skin due to sweating, and an overall increase of blood-flow to the forearm. These measures can be used to determine not only the presence of anxiety but the degree to which the subject is anxiety-prone. Some phlegmatic individuals can put up with a lot of stress before their anxiety breaks through; others, perhaps more sensitive, perhaps more imaginative, certainly more reactive, become anxious more quickly and to a greater extent.

This tendency to become anxious can also be assessed by means of questionnaires such as the Taylor Manifest Anxiety Scale, which consist of a series of questions regarding the subject's habitual response in a variety of situations, some anxiety-provoking, some not. These questionnaires require honesty of response from the subject if they are to be at all reliable and predictive, but this can be checked by the consistency of the subject's answers over a period of time and by the internal consistency of reply at any one time. Thus, what is a highly personal internal experience, and difficult to describe, can be measured and evaluated. This is vital both to research into anxiety and to assessing the treatment needed for individual patients.

Anxiety and fear are close cousins and related to a family of other words used by people suffering from phobias to describe what they are feeling. Anxiety, nervousness and worry appear to be closely related. 'I am *nervous* about going out into the shops.' 'I *worry* about having to go to the shops.' 'I become *anxious* when I think about shopping.' These statements seem to be saying the same thing: actually going out shopping, or even thinking about it, makes some people decidedly uncomfortable and distressed, to such a degree that they would prefer to avoid going out if they could.

In the same way fear, terror and panic seem to be related. 'I got such a *fright* when I went shopping and felt so awful.' 'I'm *terrified* that it will happen again if I go out.' 'I got into such a *panic* when I had to face the crowds in the shopping centre.' Here, the individual is experiencing something more dramatic and distressing in a specific setting, away from home, in the shopping precinct. Terror is acute fear which roots us to the spot; whereas panic is an acute fear which carries with it the sense of losing control and the need to take impulsive action to escape at once.

The statement 'I'm frightened to go to the shops' comes from the anticipation that something very unpleasant is going to happen which, if possible, the subject wishes to avoid. Human beings have this imaginative capacity to think forward into the future, anticipating what may happen. Anxiety is to do with the anticipatory threat of what *might*

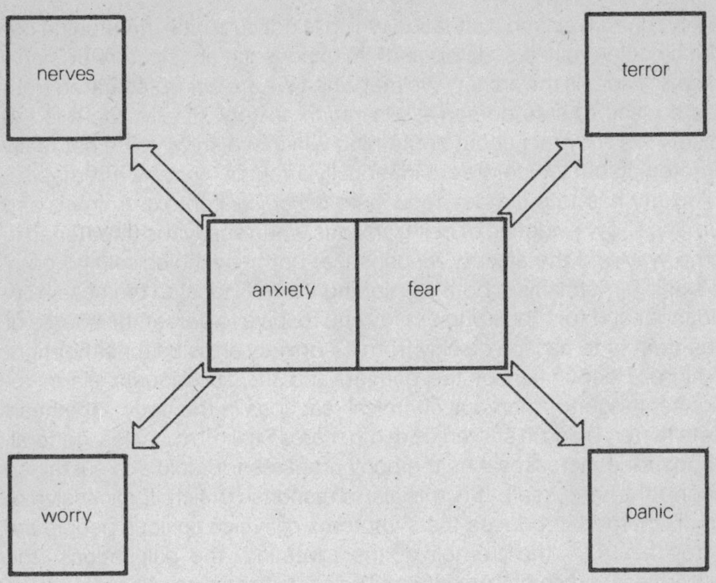

Fig. 2 Variations on a theme

happen rather than with what actually does happen. Fear, on the other hand, is what we experience when the unpleasant or dangerous is happening to us or is immediately about to happen. In common speech, anxiety and fear are often used to describe the same emotion, but one is a more acute form of the other: 'Anxiety is fear rolled out thin.' It is a matter of words, but there is no disagreement about the highly unpleasant feelings and experiences which these words are used to describe.

Anxiety comes in several forms. Very often we know exactly what we are anxious about and can say precisely what it is. This can be called *attached anxiety*, in contrast to other occasions when we feel ill-at-ease and disturbed but unable to say why. This is *free-floating anxiety*, in which the threat is coming from as much inside ourselves as from outside. It may be unresolved conflict that is troubling us, or an urge to do something of which we are ashamed and wish to disown. What is troubling us is shut away from full awareness of what it is; it may emerge later when we are more relaxed, when the conflict is resolved or on the way to resolution. At other times, we can see that we are getting ourselves into a situation which is not currently threatening but which could well be so later, and we experience anticipatory or *signal anxiety*. There is the anxiety we feel when we are being separated from a safe place or safe person – *separation anxiety*. Finally, there is the anxiety we may feel about something which we know to be not really threatening but which we are irrationally afraid of – *phobic anxiety*.

Anxiety has to be understood in its *biological context*. Animals and humans show evidence of being anxious when survival is threatened in some way and the anxiety response, at both psychological and body levels, is a mechanism both for alerting the individual to the possibility of danger and for mobilizing energy and resolve to defeat the source of the threat or to escape quickly from it – anxiety arms us for either fight or flight. Recognition of the danger, and the subsequent alarm response, trigger off nervous chemical reactions in the body – the heart beats faster, blood is shifted from other areas to limb muscles, generally body tone increases – as the body prepares for rapid and sustained action to defend itself. It is this alarm response which, if excessive or not discharged, produces the symptoms of which anxious people are all too aware – the trembling, the sweating, the palpitations, the 'butterflies' and so on. Anxiety mobilizes us to secure our selves from potential danger. Putting the anxiety and alarm response to work makes us feel better, as well as taking us away from threat.

Anxiety also plays an important part in *learning*: it sharpens our wits and strengthens our resolve to concentrate and achieve a satisfactory conclusion and reward – relief of the anxiety itself and the gaining of something pleasurable. The discomfort of moderate anxiety prompts us to discover various ways of getting away from it, and that in itself is a learning process. However, the relationship between anxiety and learning is complicated.

Increases of anxiety stimulate learning up to a certain point, beyond which further increases in anxiety bring less return, until a crucial point is reached at which more anxiety leads to a loss of learning stimulus and greater risk of errors and mistakes. This implies that there is an optimum level of anxiety for optimum learning, beyond which further rises of anxiety become counter-productive. Clinical anxiety states can now be seen as conditions in which the level of anxiety which the patient experiences is beyond this critical level, and instead of coping and dealing with problems the patient becomes distressed and disabled. If the anxiety can be brought back to the optimum level by some means, the patient has a chance of learning to be efficient once more. In its effective amount, anxiety reinforces or facilitates new learning,

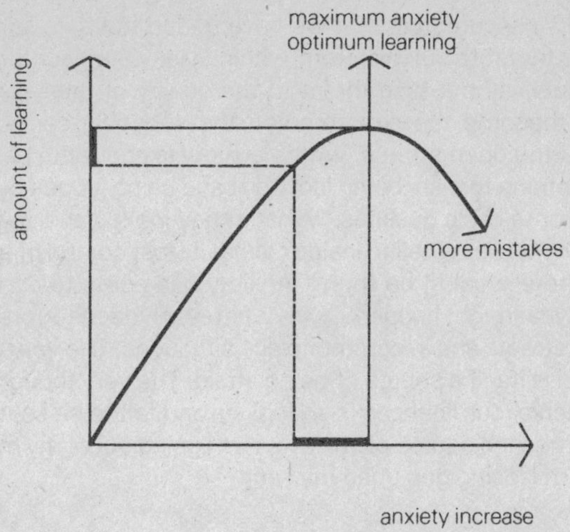

Fig. 3 Anxiety and learning

but if it is inappropriate or excessive it will reinforce and facilitate old prejudices, bad habits and disabling fears. It is a question of balance – too little and nothing happens, too much and things go wrong. In any one individual the optimum level of anxiety varies from time to time and from situation to situation, but generally people can be divided into those who operate best at a lower setting of optimum anxiety and those who operate best at a higher level. This difference is due both to inherited characteristics, and thus may run in families, and to previous learning experiences which can sensitize the person to a greater or lesser degree of anxiety.

This is the theoretical background to what happens in a phobia: anxiety levels are set, alarm responses mobilized, previous experience makes it more likely or less likely that the individual will cope. Good or bad performance sets the level for the next encounter and so on. Things get out of control, which is itself a source of further anxiety, and a vicious spiral is set up through which the sufferer progressively becomes the victim of an anxiety which is out of all proportion to the situation and which serves only to distress and disable.

Fear and physical danger go hand in hand, but in our long journey from our evolutionary past we have clambered up into a world in which, at least as far as our western culture is concerned, few have to fear for their physical survival; most have enough to get by, yet many are anxious and insecure. It is as if we have traded threat to survival from without for threat to survival from within. Many are haunted, not by a threat to survival, but by a threat to the quality of their survival. The jungle has become the supermarket, the shopping centre, the restaurant and the open streets, where anxiety is about the possibility of doing something foolish, being looked at and being judged by others as lacking in some basic qualities. 'What if they looked and saw? What if they knew what I am feeling inside? What if I lost control of myself and fainted, where would I be then?' Anxiety has come to do with what might be, what might happen – with whatever hidden terrors lie in wait in ordinary streets and in commonplace situations. The very thought of being afraid is itself a source of being afraid. The very thought of being afraid in such circumstances is so foolish, and felt to be so, that this in itself becomes the source of anxiety. 'Am I going out of my mind to feel like this? Am I losing grip upon my sanity?'

CHAPTER 2
THE ANATOMY OF A PHOBIA

A phobia is a psychological and emotional state of which phobic anxiety is the major component. Phobic anxiety is characterized by an inordinate dread of having to face or to be involved in something – the dread being out of all proportion to the degree of potential threat – together with the urge to avoid that something at all costs. It is an irrational fear which leads to avoidance behaviour. The object of fear may be other human beings, animals, places, illnesses, storms, heights, modes of travel and so on, but whatever the feared situation the resulting phobia has the following elements:

(a) The degree of anxiety and dread are out of all proportion to the situation that evokes it.
(b) They cannot be easily explained or reasoned away.
(c) They are beyond voluntary control.
(d) They lead the sufferer to avoid the feared situation as far as is possible.

Thus, people who suffer from phobias feel distressed by the condition, but also distressed, and even ashamed, because they know it is unreasonable yet cannot do anything about it. Many feel that they are being weak-minded or even that they may be going out of their minds altogether. The phobic sufferer is caught up in an endless cycle of apprehension, uncertainty, doubt and helplessness.

The degree to which the individual is aware of the phobia, and the degree to which its presence affects and limits his life, is variable. Thus, three categories can be identified:

(a) *Phobic fears*, which are so common that most people recognize they have one or other irrational fear which is part of their particular make-up. Often, these fears are of such exotic or rare objects that the individual may never, or only rarely, have to face them. A fear of snakes is very common but the chance of meeting a snake outside a zoo in western Europe is quite small.
(b) *Phobic symptoms*, in which discrete and identifiable phobic anxiety with its associated avoidance behaviour, sufficient to distress and incommode the individual, can be one of many symptoms that are part of other psychological and psychiatric states. For example, phobic anxiety may appear in states of depression and disappear when the depression is gone; it may be part of a generalized anxiety state with temporary loss of confidence; it may appear as part of the complicated rituals and avoidance behaviour of an obsessional–compulsive neurosis; finally, it can be part of serious psychiatric disorders such as a schizophrenic illness. The phobic symptom is part and parcel of

some other disorder and is symptomatic of it.

(c) *Phobic disorders*, in which phobic anxiety and avoidance are the principal features, of a nature and degree to cause immense suffering and severely limit aspects of the life and freedom of the subject, as well as those who may live with them.

Table 1 *Fears and Phobias*

Common Fears	*Phobias*
1 Universal	1 Only in certain people
2 Very frequent	2 Less frequent
3 Do not interfere with life	3 Interfere with life of patient and family
4 Tend to disappear with time	4 Do not disappear with time
5 Men and women equally affected	5 Women more often affected
6 Very common in children	6 Not common in children

Obviously, common phobic fears, being universal and usually not limiting, do not call for treatment, whereas phobic symptoms and phobic disorders do. In phobic symptoms, treatment is directed to the underlying condition; in phobic disorders treatment must focus primarily on the phobia itself.

How common are phobias? The answer to this question can be found in what are called prevalence studies, in which a given population is asked whether they experience phobic fears or actual phobic disorders. This can be done through door-to-door inquiries or by asking representative individuals to fill out detailed questionnaires from which the relevant information is subsequently extracted and evaluated. In 1897, in the USA, Stanley Hall found that a sample of 1,701 people recorded between them 6,456 fears: the most frequent was fear of thunderstorms, followed by fear of reptiles, strangers and darkness. More recently, in 1969, Agras conducted a survey of households in the Greater Burlington area of Vermont and found a prevalence rate for mild phobias (phobic fears) of 77 per thousand of the general population and for severe phobias (phobic disorders) of 2·2 per thousand. These are only average figures, and for a clearer picture his results must be looked at in some detail.

Common fears were marked in childhood but fell away in adolescence and adult life, except for the fear of death, injury, illness, separation and crowds, which continued through life. The commonest fear was of snakes (390 per thousand) and the least frequent was of being alone (44 per thousand). The pattern of *intense fears* was similar, with fear of snakes 253 per thousand and of being alone 10 per thousand. True *phobic disorders* were much less common, with fear of illness and injury 31 per thousand, and phobia for heights 4 per thousand. There were twice as many female subjects as male. Within the group, severe limiting phobic illnesses were recognized, of which 50 per cent were of leaving home and going into public places (agoraphobia), 34 per cent were of illness and injury, 8 per cent of death and of crowded places, 4 per cent of animals and 2 per cent each of heights and of the dark. Again, there were almost twice as many female sufferers as male ones.

Such studies show that phobic fears are very common and affect both males and females, and especially children. More marked phobic disorders are not common and affect females more than males.

Another way of measuring the frequency of phobic disorders is by incidence studies, that is by finding out how many phobic illnesses are represented in all the cases seen in psychiatric out-patient practices in a

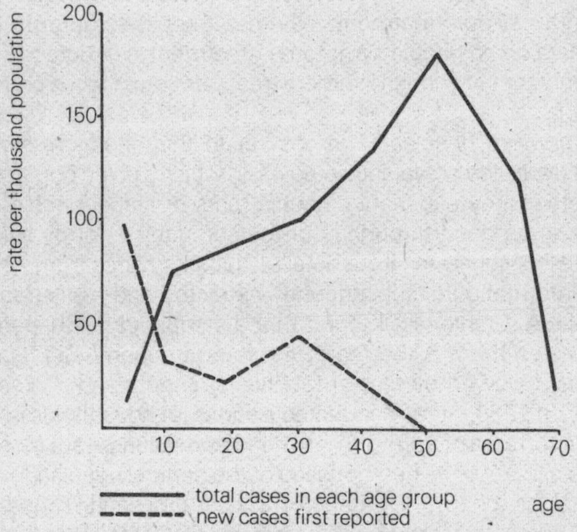

Fig. 4 Phobia trends in the general population (after Agras, 1969)

given year. In 1970, in a historical review, Marks reported that phobic disorders represented some 5 per cent of cases seen at the out-patient clinics of the Maudsley Hospital, London. In 1979, Torgersen, surveying the literature, again found that phobic disorders accounted for 2–3 per cent of all neurotic patients seen both in the USA and in Britain.

Childhood fears can be seen in young babies' natural aversion to loud noises, bright lights, sudden movements and so on. Such a startle response is quite understandable: young babies avoid anything which is strange or behaves out of the ordinary. This is a natural biological survival reaction; young babies are vulnerable and should keep away from strange situations which may well be dangerous; self-protection is paramount. Thus, it is possible that the common fear of certain animals such as snakes, dogs and large predators is a racial memory from times when such animals could threaten the survival of human beings in the wild.

However, that the response of babies to potential danger is more subtle and immediate than this is shown by an experiment called the 'visual cliff'. A sheet of stout glass is placed over a clearly defined drop, painted in black and white squares. A child at the crawling and curious stage is put on to the glass. The child will crawl over the glass as long as there is firm ground immediately beneath, but when it comes to the visual cliff-edge it will go no further, even though driven by curiosity it *could* do so, supported by the glass. Long before the child can form the concepts 'height', 'fall' and 'hurt', by instinct as it were, it will not put itself at risk, although it knows it is supported by the glass above the drop. In such an experiment, many children are reluctant even to crawl anywhere near the drop, which suggests that human beings may have inherent avoidance patterns which are essentially of survival value. Fear of strangers (xenophobia), although capable of later political and racist interpretations, may well have a similar origin.

Common fears in childhood reach their peak at about three or four years of age, when otherwise quite normal children will become frightened even with their parents present. Their sleep is haunted by terrifying nightmares. Most of these fears recede as the children grow older, but a study by Abe in Osaka, Japan, showed that of 242 mothers of frightened children, of those mothers who themselves in childhood showed marked fear of thunder, animals or injections, 35 per cent were still suffering these same fears as adults. Agras's study in Vermont showed that fears of death, injury, illness and separation in crowds may well persist from childhood into adult life.

Adult fears are many but they can be classified under five headings:

(a) *separation fears* of being alone and unaccompanied either at home or, more commonly, in public; of being left alone in places such as the hospital or the dentist.
(b) *animal fears* of all kinds – snakes, birds, spiders, cats, dogs, horses, bats, insects, mice, etc.
(c) *mutilation fears* of being hurt by doctors or dentists, of being cut, of knives and axes, of any sharp object, of blood, of losing parts of the body, of being disfigured in some way.
(d) *social fears* such as being unable to go unaccompanied into shops, theatres and churches; being unable to eat in a restaurant for fear of vomiting or making a fool of oneself; being terrified of having to speak in public or having to act in front of others.
(e) *nature fears* such as fear of thunderstorms, strong winds, fire, heights, deep water, mountains, waterfalls, wide-open spaces and so on.

All these fears are theoretically understandable because they refer to some state of danger, discomfort or self-consciousness, but the degree of dread is unreasonable and leads to a greater or lesser tendency to avoidance.

How do such common fears come about? In human terms there is rarely one cause for anything, and complex behaviour is built up from a variety of antecedent factors. Anxiety and fear, although distressing, have a protective and motivating function. Thus, many common fears may stem from our much more immediately physically dangerous past, where survival from day to day depended upon eternal vigilance and awareness of potential dangers around. Such fears therefore may represent our *evolutionary past* inside us.

Many fears are *cultural* in that they are taught, sometimes consciously, often unconsciously, to each other. Unfortunate events occur and generalizations are made from these specifics. Rumours and myths circulate, and attitudes are pre-formed. Certain people, certain circumstances, are declared dangerous and to be avoided if at all possible. Prejudice is perpetuated by gossip and anecdotal tales. People learn to be afraid, expect to be afraid and thus prepare themselves to be afraid, and becoming afraid prove to themselves how right the tales of others were. Fear becomes a self-fulfilling prophecy. Other fears are consciously manipulated by others for political, racist or financial advantage. For every human anxiety there is a remedy offered, but usually at a price.

Some people, because of their *personalities*, are going to be more liable to fears than others. The anxious individual is already prepared to be anxious in most situations. Obsessional, precise people get upset when they feel that they are losing control of what is going on around them, and worry about it. Vulnerable dependent personalities will always want someone to be with them, to take over and protect them if things get difficult. Suspicious, threatened people see danger all around and expect to be hurt and rejected. There is, however, no evidence for a specific phobic personality. Anxiety, fear and phobia can build up in anyone, although some are more susceptible than others.

Social factors also play a part. People are apt to feel more isolated and threatened in large anonymous urban environments than elsewhere. Family units are smaller and often separated from supportive relatives. With growing tension between racial groups, economic uncertainty and the rise of violence in the larger cities people are becoming alienated from each other and from themselves. In 1956, Tucker, in a study of phobic disorders in Boston, showed that phobias were more likely in women than in men, in young wives and mothers than in older women, and in the married than in the single, especially in those with dependent, anxious personalities.

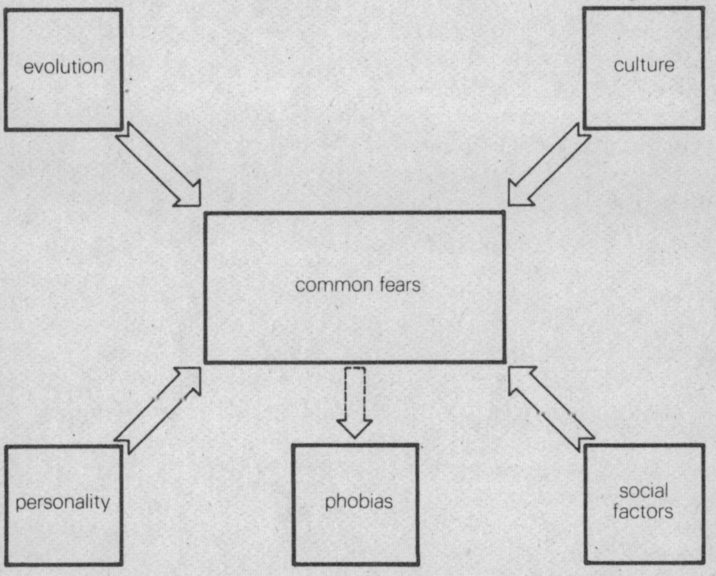

Fig. 5 Origins of fears and phobias

Common fears, to which many are prone, can therefore be the base-line from which true phobias start to evolve later because of the intervention of other factors.

CHAPTER 3
VARIETIES OF PHOBIC ILLNESSES

Phobic fears are common, especially in children, but in adults, although a cause for concern to the individual, they rarely result in avoidance behaviour of such a degree as to disturb people's lives. They know that there are things and situations which they would rather avoid if at all possible, but life goes on as usual.

Phobic symptoms are frequently found in association with other psychiatric states and add to the overall distress and disability from which the patient suffers. In a survey in Newcastle made in 1979, of 102 alcoholics admitted to a special alcoholic unit 30 per cent suffered from disabling agoraphobias or social phobias and a further 30 per cent had similar but less disabling symptoms. In a previous Newcastle study, 111 patients admitted to hospital between 1963 and 1965 because of affective illnesses (depression or anxiety) showed evidence of associated phobic symptoms. Patients with anxiety states were found to have significantly more phobias both before and during their illness than patients with depression. Specific phobias (precise fears) were relatively unaffected by illness, whereas the degree of social phobias and agoraphobias were frequently related to it.

Phobic disorders sufficient to disturb and disrupt the life-style of the individual patient and the family are relatively rare, perhaps affecting some 10–20 per thousand of the general population. Although relatively uncommon, true phobic disorders are nevertheless very distressing to the sufferer and to family relatives – whole families may be disturbed, especially if the mother is the one affected.

In 1970, Marks made a ten-year retrospective study of all the patients seen at the Maudsley Hospital, London, who were diagnosed as suffering from a phobic disorder. He divided these into phobic illnesses of external origin, in which the source of the phobic anxiety lay outside the patient, and those of internal origin, in which the distress arose from fears about the integrity of the self (Table 2).

Table 2 *Origins of phobias*

	Type	*Frequency*
Phobias of external origin	agoraphobia	60 per cent
	misc. specific phobias	14 per cent
	social phobias	8 per cent
	animal phobias	3 per cent

Phobias of internal origin:	illness phobias obsessional phobias (re-classified)	15 per cent

Agoraphobia was the commonest and in some ways the most distressing illness seen. It occurs mostly in women, with symptoms beginning after puberty and prominent from fifteen to thirty-five years of age. It is rare in childhood. Phobic anxiety centres on leaving home to go out into public places and is accompanied by signs of severe anxiety levels such as tension, dizziness, panic and unreality feelings. The illness shows a fluctuating course and can be seen as a discrete and coherent syndrome with a well-defined cluster of symptoms. As this is the most common phobic illness, it will be described in more detail later.

Miscellaneous specific phobias (monosymptomatic phobias) centre round specifically feared and avoided experiences: heights, strong winds, thunderstorms, darkness, running water, enclosed spaces and so on. These illnesses can start at any time in life and persist throughout life. They affect men and women equally. A young married man woke one night to find the roof of his garden shed being blown off in a gale. He was alarmed at the time, but not particularly frightened; however, he thereafter found himself assiduously watching the weather forecasts for hint of storms and becoming irrationally worked up whenever there was a chance of high winds. He could not sleep for worrying, went off his food, began to lose weight and became quite depressed. A married woman was always afraid of enclosed spaces, but it did not interfere with her life. One day, in a large department store, she had a panic attack in the lift. Now she will not go into large shops and has recurring nightmares about being trapped in dark holes. Her husband is losing all patience with her because she cannot tell him what it is all about, and he thinks she is behaving in this way deliberately to annoy him.

Social phobias are concerned with terrors of having to eat or drink in public, of blushing in mixed company, of having to speak or to write in front of others. There is no inherent fear of crowds as such, as there is in agoraphobia, but only of making a fool of oneself in front of other people in some particular way. Such phobias begin at puberty, with an upsurge in adolescence, and in adult life they merge, in effect, into agoraphobia but are less coherent entities. They have to be disting-

…om simple shyness or social awkwardness by the degree of … and the recognized irrationality of the fears. There is a small …oup of people who are socially accident-prone; they cause as much embarrassment to others as to themselves, as they stumble from one social mishap to another. A competent secretary found herself blushing when a personable young man came into the office. The other girls pulled her leg about it. She thought no more about it until she found herself worrying that she might blush again, especially with her boss. She began blushing in all kinds of inappropriate situations, so that she now cannot go into work because of her embarrassment and thinks she may be going mad. A rather precise and fastidious professional man who lives on his own used to enjoy eating out at restaurants of his choice. He thought of himself as rather a gourmet. One day he had the irresistible fear that he was going to be sick in the restaurant in front of all the other diners; he rushed from the room and has not been able to go out to eat since. He is furious with what he sees as his weakness, but can neither explain it nor do anything about it.

Animal phobias are the most clear-cut but the least common phobic disorders. Many of them start in childhood, as young as three or four years of age, and persist throughout life. Men and women are equally affected. Almost any animal can be feared to an irrational degree, but many are household pets or domestic animals – cats, dogs, guinea pigs, mice, rats, horses; others are relatively rare, such as snakes, worms or bats. An irrational fear of fluttering birds, or even fluttering moths, is not uncommon, as is fear of certain insects – bees, wasps, and especially spiders and earwigs. The fear is out of all proportion to the real danger which the animal may represent. Such phobias cause untold suffering and can imprison the sufferer within the home lest a feared animal is encountered in the garden or in the street outside. Because such a phobia is so discrete, it often carries the best hope for treatment.

Illness phobias. Many patients, although they know that there is no rational basis for such a belief, are nevertheless haunted by an overwhelming fear that they have a cancer, a heart disease, or an infection such as tuberculosis. Others know they do not have any serious disease, yet have a paralysing presentiment that they are about to die. Such patients ruminate on the possibility of crippling or of fatal illnesses, while at the same time saying, 'I know it's stupid, but this is how I feel, and I can't get away from it. It's driving me and my family out of our minds.' Men and women are equally affected, and these phobias can come on at any age in adolescence and adult life. Their course is erratic and they are often made worse by concurrent depression or by episodes of acute anxiety. Such patients are not hypochondriacal, in that they know on one level that they are not ill, yet on another suffer as if they were. The true hypochondriac is quite convinced that he is ill and may even enjoy it. Neither are the phobic victims malingerers who choose to pretend to be ill for some hidden gain or purpose.

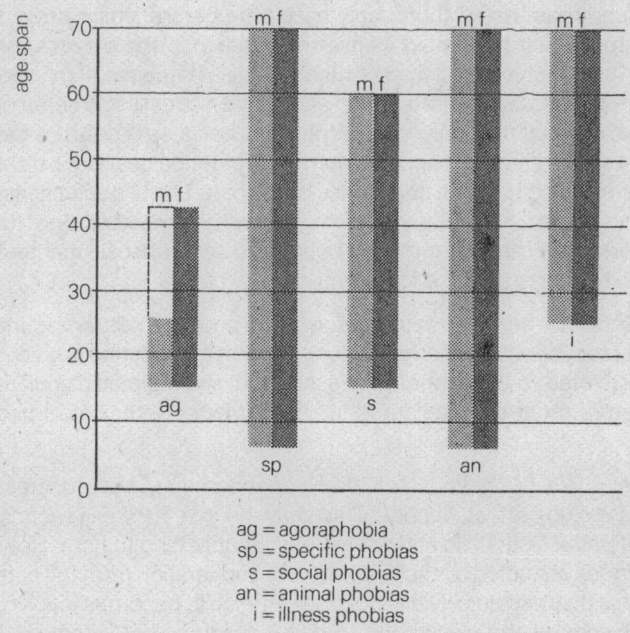

Fig. 6 Clinical problems

Obsessional phobias, so called, are now classified as obsessional disorders and are not considered to be true phobias, although they share certain 'phobic' qualities – the fear is disproportionate to the situation, it cannot be explained away and it is beyond voluntary control. Such disorders are characterized by a persistent fear of having caused harm to others by some unforgivable negligence; some small act is blown up out of all proportion and is believed to have caused irreparable harm to others. A man believed that, as he was driving along, a piece of paper touched his exhaust pipe, caught alight and was blown onto a house, setting it on fire. He was convinced that he had caused the deaths of the inhabitants. The incident did not actually occur, but he is continually tormented by the idea that it may have and that he is to blame. He searches the streets for evidence of houses set on fire as his car was passing. Other patients believe that they can hand on some infection or disease to the family; thus all crockery and utensils must be scrupulously washed in disinfectant each day to prevent contamination. One man believed that he had picked up a germ from handling coins, and must bathe thoroughly each time before sitting down to a family meal, lest he should inadvertently pass on the disease to the others by touching a dish or brushing against their cutlery. These bizarre illnesses, which affect men and women equally and come on at any age, are best not considered as phobias, because the sufferer fears not that something will happen to him – the criterion of all phobias – but to *others*, owing to some negligence on his part. There is an obsessional conviction of guilt, derived from an over-valued idea, and these disorders therefore have more in common with obsessional states, especially their resistance to treatment.

While these are the main groupings of phobic disorders found in clinical practice, five other conditions have been described which are closely related to these phobic illnesses and, sharing many similarities with them, must be considered in any survey of pathological phobic states.

School phobia. Many young children are apprehensive and distressed on first being left at school. This may be the first experience of separation for both child and parent, and be upsetting to both. However, if properly handled by the teacher, with cooperation from the parent, this initial distress quickly disappears as the child becomes involved in the activities of the classroom. In some children this separation distress continues and, because the child seems to be afraid of being at school, the condition has been loosely labelled 'school phobia', but it is now known as 'school refusal' to indicate that, although the clinical picture is similar, it is not a true phobia. The separation anxiety and the uncertainty about fitting in with strange teachers and with schoolfellows are understandable, if undesirable. Further, the children are normally not avoiding school as such, but are trying to avoid separation from home and parents. The school is only the context within which the separation is experienced.

Baker and Willis, from Staffordshire, reported in 1978 a group of ninety-nine cases of school refusal seen at a child-guidance clinic over a period of twelve years. They divided the children into two groups: an acute group which contained the youngest children, with two or less brothers or sisters, with somewhat older mothers; and a chronic group comprising children of all ages, from larger families, with younger mothers. These children conformed to the criteria first described by Berg in 1969:

(a) severe difficulty in attending school leading to prolonged absence
(b) severe emotional upset with increased fearfulness, temper tantrums, unhappiness and a tendency to complain of symptoms without any objective signs, especially just before setting off for school
(c) remaining at home with the knowledge and agreement of the parents
(d) absence of any significant antisocial behaviour seen in other disturbed children such as lying, stealing or destructiveness

In 1976, Berg, in a study of 125 adolescents followed up for seven years after treatment for school refusal, showed that one third improved substantially or completely, one third improved to a degree but now showed other symptoms, and one third remained seriously affected. Thus, a substantial number of children can be expected to grow out of this disorder in time. The indicators of a poorer result in Berg's study were high intelligence plus an inadequate response to treatment at the time of discharge from in-patient care.

In another study in 1976 Berg showed that school refusal occurred to a greater extent than expected in children with mothers who were themselves agoraphobic, 14 per cent of their children showing the disorder in the age-group eleven to fifteen years. Many of the agoraphobic mothers had themselves suffered from school refusal. Berg surveyed 786 women members of an agoraphobic correspondence club and found that those mothers who themselves had suffered from school refusal had experienced an earlier onset of agoraphobia and had a greater tendency to have children who would suffer from school refusal.

Eisenberg, in Baltimore in 1958, had already shown that in twenty-six children suffering from school refusal there was an over-dependence on the parents, which had been fostered by the parents because of their own emotional needs. The mothers were themselves anxious and indecisive, having had a poor relationship with their own mothers. The parents' anxious attitudes appeared to be transferred to the children and provides a good example of learned fearfulness.

Travel phobias. Many adults are terrified of flying, and to a certain extent this is understandable even though it is well known that flying is the safest means of transport per passenger mile. In reality, there may not be much chance of survival if the plane does crash. But other adults are equally frightened of travelling by bus, ship or even family car in circumstances where most people, even if they know the real risks involved, are not unduly concerned. In a true travel phobia, an individual is excessively afraid of travelling in a certain way which most other people would accept without concern. Some travellers are frightened of missing a connection and deliberately arrive early to be certain of not doing so; others are terrified that they will be carried beyond their destination and will be unable to get off the vehicle in time; others feel shut in and sick (claustrophobia); some are plagued by motion sickness; others feel anxious about abandoning themselves to the skill of the driver, the pilot or captain and, like obsessionals, are uneasy about giving up control of themselves and their destiny to others. For some the phobia may be the crowds or open spaces, as in agoraphobia; for others it may resemble the separation anxiety of school refusal – an enforced separation, albeit for a time only, from loved ones or from the safety of mother earth. Travel phobia is thus not a single condition but the end result of a large number of contributory factors.

Phobic depersonalization syndrome was first described by Roth in 1959. Sufferers experience a combination of acute phobic anxiety and a particularly disturbing sensation called 'depersonalization'. They feel as if a cloud is coming down over the level of their self-consciousness: they feel unpleasantly detached, as if they are observing themselves from the outside; they feel as if they are about to come apart in some way and see it as the sign of incipient madness. Such patients Roth described as dependent, scrupulous, fastidious and rigid in outlook (again, rather like obsessionals, fearing loss of control). In some of the patients this condition had come on after some tragedy or severe stress and was thought to be a calamity reaction, but such an antecedent was not always present. Roth found that 40 per cent had detectable abnormalities in the nervous system and thought that the condition might reflect some underlying brain defect. However, this condition is now known to occur in the absence of brain disease and is due to a high level of circulating noradrenaline, the alarm chemical released into the bloodstream in the face of imminent danger. Why depersonalization should occur with phobic anxiety in some patients and not with others remains unclear.

Housebound housewives. In 1964, Roberts, from St George's Hospital, London, described thirty-eight married women who were imprisoned in their homes by phobic anxiety and associated attacks of panic. They were in the age-range of twenty to forty years and had experienced a sudden onset with a severe disabling and distressing panic attack. He found that in their personalities they were anxiety-prone, somewhat obsessional and rather tense individuals. The description of the woman as a prisoner in her own home is a dramatic one but it is exactly what many phobics fear most. Again, it is not a single condition but the end result of a number of phobic illnesses and separation anxiety. Women with agoraphobia, social phobias, animal phobias and illness phobias can end up imprisoned at home if they become so frightened that they dare not go out even if accompanied by someone. This is an example of extreme avoidance behaviour. Other housebound women are suffering less from a real phobia than from severe separation anxiety: they are afraid to leave home rather than afraid of what waits for them in the world outside.

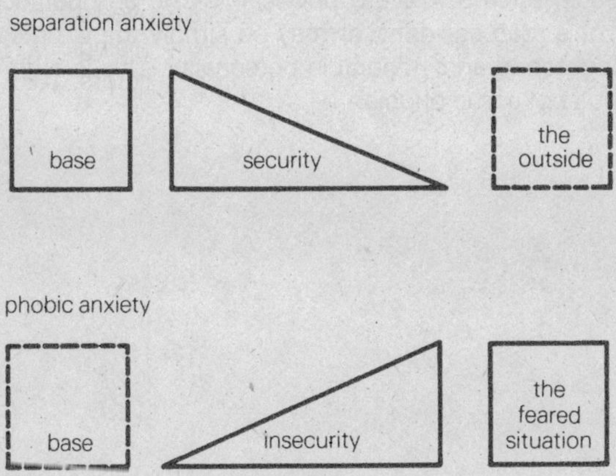

Fig. 7 Separation and phobic anxieties

In *separation anxiety* there would appear to be a logical sequence:

(a) I am frightened to be on my own, for then I will be away from someone dependable, someone who knows me well.

(b) This realization is making my heart beat fast and I can't breathe so well: this makes me feel worse.

(c) If I am on my own, I may not be able to get in touch with someone to help me – I would have to cope on my own. I don't think I can, while I feel as awful as this.
(d) I feel trapped and want to shout 'help', but I don't know in what way I want help; this makes me feel stupid as well as afraid. I know all this is irrational, but I can't help it, and that makes me feel embarrassed and very cross with myself.
(e) All this makes me feel as if something awful is going to happen to me, but I don't know what. I'm frightened, I'm trapped, I'm terrified. Whatever can I do? Whatever will people think of me?

Thus, there is a sense of 'being on one's own' together with an inability to close the gap between the self and the security base.

Pan-phobic reaction is the last state of mind to be considered. Here the individual is frightened not of anything specific, or even of a group of related objects or events, but of everything; everything is seen as a danger. This reflects a generalized anxiety and generalized loss of self-confidence, of self-autonomy, which may be due to an overwhelming occurrence, such as severe physical illness, an operation, a bereavement or a road accident, or may be simply the expression of a habitually frightened and vulnerable personality. This is a generalized state and thus not a true phobia.

CHAPTER 4
AGORAPHOBIA

Agoraphobia is the most frequent form of phobic disorder encountered – constituting 60 per cent of all phobias seen at the Maudsley Hospital, London, over ten years and affecting approximately some six per thousand of the general population. It is a puzzling and intriguing condition, which has been recognized clinically for over a hundred years. In 1870, Benedikt, in an Austrian medical journal, described a disorder which he called *Platzschwindel*, or dizziness in public places. He emphasized the unpleasant bodily effects which the patient experienced. In 1872, Westphal published a monograph entitled *Die Agoraphobie*, in which were described three male patients suffering from an inability to walk through certain streets and public squares without a resultant dread and profound anxiety, and without fear of loss of consciousness. The anticipatory dread was worst when the streets were empty and the shops shut. The patients were comforted if they could be accompanied by a friend, or even supported by a cane or a vehicle of some sort. Westphal noted that in one of his patients the fear of sparsely built-up streets in town was greater than his fear of the open countryside, and another had the greatest difficulty in crossing a bridge over running water.

The word 'agoraphobia' comes from two roots – *agora* and *phobos*. The *agora* was the public meeting-place of the Greek city states which, because of the hot Mediterranean climate, was out in the open air or in the market place. Thus it was the public place for meeting one's friends and for doing business. In our modern northern European context it has the connotations of shopping, business and any social transaction taking place in the streets, shopping precincts and in public buildings such as banks, cinemas, theatres or churches. Phobos was a Greek god who could strike acute fear and panic into the hearts of his enemies, and thus a phobia is an acute fear or panic state of irrational origins.

Thus, agoraphobia has come to mean an overwhelming fear or dread of going out into public areas where business is transacted or people meet. It has lost much of the original nineteenth-century sense of fear of open spaces as such. Some patients are terrified of being on their own in wide-open spaces, such as fields or deserted moorland, but in this they are similar to people who are afraid to be left alone anywhere and are probably suffering from a form of separation anxiety, being afraid that something unpleasant will happen to them because there is no one there who could come to their aid.

If agoraphobia means literally a fear of going out into public places where there is a busy throng of people, claustrophobia – a fear of being trapped in a confined space – could well be a component. This is just what many anxious patients fear most: a terror of being caught in the check-out queue at the supermarket as they have to wait to pay for their trolley load, or of being in a cinema or theatre audience, or in a church, from which they cannot easily escape. To try to rush out would be socially undesirable, serving only to attract unwelcome attention. Such people always try to sit at the back, or at least at the end of a row, from which they hope they can make a discreet departure if the occasion calls for it. They are not physically trapped, as in a true claustrophobia, but held captive by convention and social expectation: they could leave the check-out queue, they could leave the church, but to do so only draws attention to their plight, and they anticipate others will disapprove or even be frankly hostile to them.

With common usage over time, the term agoraphobia has come to be applied to a rather vague collection of situational fears, the essence

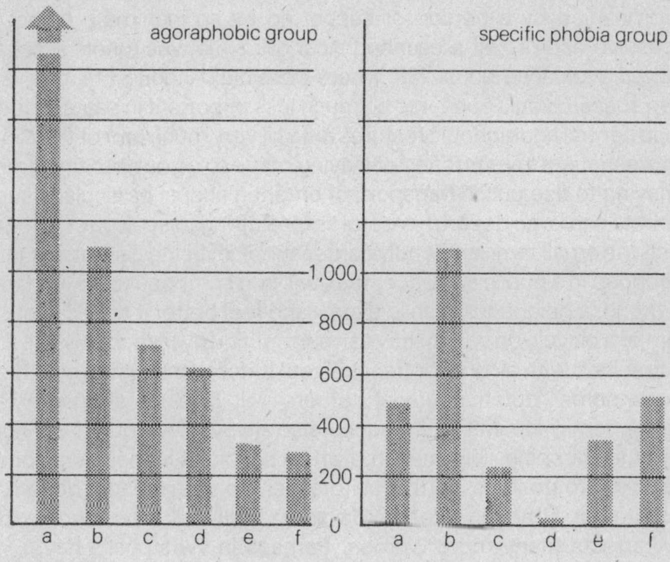

a = going away from home
b = travelling
c = traffic
d = being alone
e = crowds
f = eating in public

Fig. 8. Percentage increases in fear score before and after onset of illness (after Snaith, 1968)

of which involves leaving the security of home to go out into the public streets. In 1968, Snaith published a detailed survey of specific phobias compared to agoraphobias. He used a 'fear schedule', in which the people interviewed were asked to rate themselves against a list of forty common fears, grading the degree of fear against a four-point scale. He then calculated the increase in fear rating before and after the onset of illness in two groups of patients – the first with agoraphobia, the second with a primary fear focused on some object or situation.

The agoraphobic group is characterized by fear of leaving home and of travelling (presumably away from home), whereas group two is afraid of travelling itself and of eating in public, although it did not like to be away from home either. The agoraphobic group was afraid of crowds and of wide-open spaces, but to a very much lesser extent.

The principal symptoms of Westphal's original three patients were a fear and dread of walking in public streets and squares, relief if accompanied by a person or supported by an inanimate object, an excessive use of self-prescribed alcoholic sedatives (beer, wine) and marked avoidance behaviour where possible. Although fear of wide-open spaces would appear to be much less important in patients today, these central agoraphobic features are still very much part of the clinical picture. Patients are terrified of leaving home to go out into the streets, of having to use public transport, of entering shops, particularly supermarkets and large department stores (preferring to seek out, if they still exist, the small familiar friendly corner shop), of being caught in queues or trapped in a public audience; they will beg someone to go with them – a friend, a neighbour, a child even – and feel better if they can push a pram or a bicycle on which they can surreptitiously lean; many will dose themselves with alcohol or tranquillizers beforehand just to give themselves some 'dutch courage'; others will give up altogether and arrange family life so that someone else always goes out of the home to do the shopping. They become virtual prisoners in their own homes, having to forgo trips to the hairdresser, to the theatre or to local restaurants. Although Westphal's cases were all men, agoraphobia now affects many more women. Perhaps in Westphal's day it was unfashionable for ladies to discuss such things with male doctors, but today the convention is reversed in that it may be easier for wives and mothers to go to the family doctor shyly to confess to such fears, whereas it might be thought unmanly for husbands and fathers so to do. On the other hand, men and women equally report specific situational or animal phobias, so that a true sexual bias may exist in the agoraphobic syndrome.

In his survey, Snaith found that the onset of the agoraphobia was quite variable: in some it was sudden, arising out of an overwhelming anxiety or panic; in others it came on slowly and imperceptibly. In a few, it was erratic, with several small episodes of isolated attacks of anxiety or panic before the onset of the major disorder, with its sustained pattern of phobic anxiety and avoidance behaviour. Characteristically, this condition comes on after puberty, and many patients say it first appeared, as far as they can remember, after marriage or after the birth of the first child. Are these true causal links or are they merely sign-posts in the life history of the individual patient against which the onset of the illness is registered? Most patients cannot understand why they have become as they are, often saying that they have nothing really to worry about but that it is all very perplexing and upsetting.

A family doctor referring an agoraphobic patient to a psychiatrist for assessment might write of 'this pleasant married woman with a young family, who has no previous history of psychiatric illness. She is very much a sensible and effective wife and mother, but recently she has been prone to panic attacks when she is out of the home. These are sufficiently distressing to interfere with her life, in that she can no longer go shopping or visit her friends. She and her husband are at a loss to understand what is causing all this. Although initially she felt better on the sedatives which I prescribed for her, they are no longer effective. I will be grateful if you would see her and suggest what can be done to help her.'

On taking a full history, it is confirmed that the patient, although on occasions a little shy, has always managed to cope with her life very well. However, after the birth of her first child she became more anxious and less competent, and then one day after the birth of the second, for no apparent reason, had a severe panic attack while standing in the check-out queue at the supermarket. She felt hot and sweaty, and was terrified that she might faint. Her husband had to take her home, and thereafter even the thought of going out shopping has caused her distress, she has tried, but even though she was accompanied by her husband, the panic feelings came back, although not so severely. During the attack, she feels distant from herself and cannot think clearly. She feels that she is about to pass out, though she does not do so. If anyone speak to her, she knows what she wants to say, but her mind goes blank, or the words come out in such a jumble that she feels so embarrassed, which only makes her feel much worse. Not unnaturally, she begins to wonder if she is going out of her mind, and rather than expose herself to such experiences, which she is now convinced will happen every time, she prefers to remain at home with the children, sending her husband and her mother to do the shopping. By this stage, she has forgotten, if she ever knew, what caused the panic in the first place, and now she is convinced the same thing will happen whenever she leaves home and so does not put it to the test. The fear has become established and certain, as well as her own sense of frustration and helplessness.

While Westphal, in his classical description of the illness, put emphasis on the fear of open spaces as the primary defect, the modern view of agoraphobia sees it as a complex pattern of behaviour in which there is no one specific fear; rather there is a cluster of fears related to leaving the security of the home to go out into public places. Crowds of people, loud noises, busy public transport, all convey to the agoraphobic a sense of being overwhelmed, with a subsequent fear of helplessness. There is an associated fear of loss of control, leading to the possibility of some act which might draw attention to the self, with increased shame

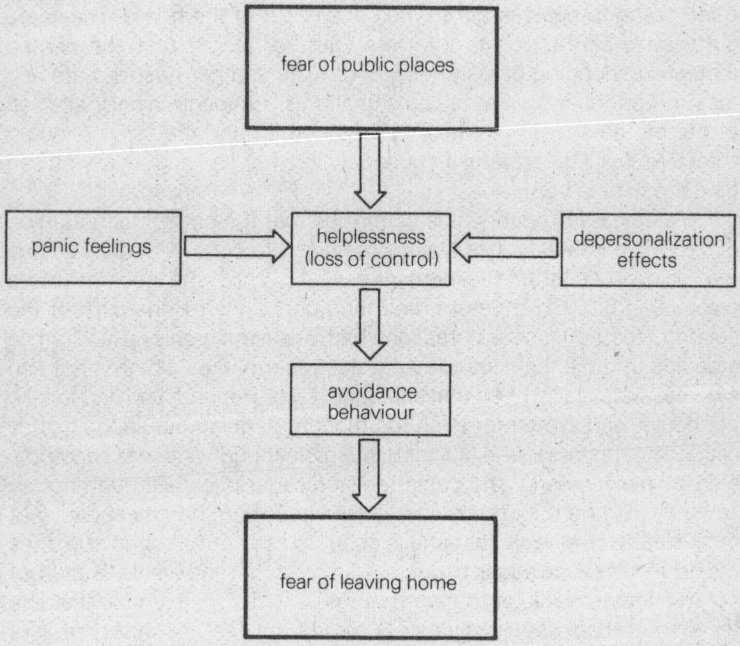

Fig. 9 The agoraphobic syndrome

and guilt. There is generalized loss of confidence and exaggeration of dependency traits, as the individual gives up responsibility for the self and abandons it to others. Life activities become progressively restricted, and the patient is ultimately imprisoned within the confines of their own fearfulness.

Thus, agoraphobia is different from other situational or specific phobias in that agoraphobic patients are generally more anxious, and fearful of a constellation of related situations – leaving home, travelling, traffic, crowds, being alone and so on. In many ways this disorder is closer to the concept of separation anxiety than to phobic anxiety, in that leaving the safety and security of home or of a companion exposes a secondary fear of being in shops, crowds and so on, rather than a primary irrational fear of these shops and crowds themselves. The patient is aware of the fear of shops and not so aware of the more basic fear of separation. This has led some authors to question the validity of the classic name of agoraphobia for this condition in modern times, and to suggest some other but less telling name such as 'non-specific insecurity reaction' or 'separation anxiety syndrome'. However, the condition is so common and the old name used so often that it is likely to remain in common usage for quite a time to come.

CHAPTER 5
WHAT CAUSES PHOBIAS?

Making a detailed description of the varieties of different phobic disorders is relatively easy: saying what brings them about is not. Apart from the distress inherent in the condition itself, not knowing what has caused it adds much to the plight of phobic sufferers. For nearly all patients the illness remains a mystery: 'Why has it happened to me, why at this time of my life when everything seems otherwise to be going well? I know it doesn't make sense, so why does it persist when I'm trying to break away from it?'

Any explanation for such a disorder has to account for the timing of its onset, why particular people are affected, why it is so irrational and why the behaviour pattern persists while the individual is struggling against it. Some explanations are offered, which can be classified into four major groups: psychodynamic explanations based on psychological theories of the mind; behavioural explanations based on learning theories of neurological function; ethological and social explanations based on animal and human acts in groups; and finally individual explanations which patients work out for themselves but find perhaps not altogether convincing.

Why press for explanations? Because not to know, to remain in doubt and uncertainty, is itself distressing and a source of secondary anxiety. As human beings we want to know, and need to know, why we behave in the way we do. Only then can we have any sense of mastery and control over our destinies. If the patient knows why he has a phobia, he is that nearer to doing something about it. Sometimes knowing does not lead to change, but at least ambiguity is dealt with. Thus it is worth looking in some detail at each of the four groups of explanations for phobic behaviour.

(1) Psychodynamic explanations

One of the functions of the mind is to assimilate experience and to make sense of it, to attribute meaning to it, because out of meaning comes a sense of order and understanding, which in turn gives a sense of mastery and control. The mind deals with perceptions which lead to thoughts, and to feelings about these thoughts. When something happens to us we see what is happening, which produces thoughts, which give rise to the appropriate feelings. This triad of perception, thought and feeling is then compared with a vast library of previous experiences, and some glimmer of meaning begins to emerge. The quality of our previous experiences enables us to make some sense of our present ones.

The building-bricks of the mind are sense data derived from neurological activity in the brain. These sense data are organized into symbols which carry meaning and feeling; it is these symbols which are manipulated by the mind in 'understanding' what is happening to us. This is difficult to grasp, and an illustration may help. To get round the London Underground, most of us use small maps made up of different-coloured lines for the various routes and coloured dots for the stations. This map bears very little resemblance to the real Underground system, but is a symbol of it. The map contains the essence of the Underground system in terms of connections between one station and the next, so that we can use this symbolic representation (the map) to find our way round the Underground (external reality). A detailed 'true' representational plan of the actual Underground system would be too large and confusing, and have too much information, for us to make proper and practical use of it; it would probably get us lost. The symbolic representation is clearer and to the point, and has enough information for our needs. So the mind reduces the reality of the external world into a inner map of symbols which it uses to find its way, as it tries to make some sense of what is happening in the outside world. Each of us therefore lives in two worlds: the external world of public reality, and the internal world of symbolic personal private reality. The mind mediates between each. With phobias, the question is: are we afraid of the literal external and public world, or does our fear arise from the inner world of symbols which is projected as it were outwards onto the screen of the external world? In other words, is the agoraphobic afraid of the actual streets and shops, or does the fear arise out of the internal world of symbolic representations of those streets and shops inside the mind?

We have had to come by a somewhat difficult route to arrive at this point, but the essence of psychodynamic explanations for phobias, which sets them aside from all other explanations, is this assumption – that the fear originates in the inner private world and is then projected outwards onto the public world of others. This explanation is only a hypothesis, and cannot be proved in a scientific sense. It is itself a kind of map. All that can be asked of it is: does this explanation (this map) help us to find our way about the phobias?

Many of Freud's early ideas about anxiety, and phobic anxiety in particular, were revised by him in an important case study, 'Analysis of a Phobia in a Five-Year-Old Boy', published in 1909. The boy has come to be known as Little Hans, and Freud's paper covers the story of events between 1906 and 1908, when Hans was three to five years old. Freud did not meet Hans himself regularly, but received reports from Hans's father, a physician and follower of Freud's method. The story tells how Hans becomes afraid of horses – especially of horses biting or falling down in the street. His concern was sparked off after he had witnessed one horse urinating in a field, and another, pulling a public bus, which fell down in the road and kicked its legs in the air, as if it was dying. Thereafter, Hans became irrationally afraid of horses, and as these were quite common at the time in Vienna, where he lived, this had a considerable effect on the boy and on his family. Could this fear be understood? Freud comments that Hans is a cheerful and forward child and not particularly nervous, but like all children of his age he is caught up in complicated feelings about his parents. He is rather afraid of his somewhat distant father and very fond of his mother: he wants to be close to her all the time, but she spends time with his father when he comes home. Hans becomes jealous of his father, and in his imagination plots to get rid of him so that he can have his mother all to himself. Hans realizes that his father will sense that this is how he feels and will want to punish Hans for having such wicked thoughts. Hans now becomes afraid of his father, but what is the connection with horses? It is a question of symbolic similarity. Father is large, strong and powerful, just as horses are to a little boy. Hans is caught up in an emotional conflict: he loves his father, but wants to get rid of him; father is a rival and must be 'killed off' in imagination. The fear of the biting horse contains the fear of the punishing father, and just as the horse fell down 'as if it were dying', so might his father die if Hans were to wish it so. Then he would be full of guilt, so that being afraid of the horse protects him from conscious fear of his father, and the horse can be finished off in his mind, as a symbolic substitute for his father. Thus, the internal danger (the punishing father) is transformed into an external danger (the biting horse). Neurotic anxiety, arising out of the original conflict of loving and envying, is turned into a more acceptable anxiety about a particular type of animal.

Using such a model of explanation, psychodynamic theory would identify the original inner conflict, a dynamic struggle between what we want for ourselves and what we ought to forgo for the sake of others, and to see how this is displaced outwards onto a substitute external object. We can fly from an external danger by consciously avoiding it; we cannot so easily escape from a danger arising out of a conflict deep inside us. Thus agoraphobics are seen as people who are afraid of the impulses aroused in them by those they meet in the street. Early analyses of agoraphobics revealed the street as a symbolic opportunity for sexual adventures. What such patients are afraid of, says the theory, is that they will give way to sexual temptation and thus be the focus of public disapproval and rejection. The original conflict – the wish to be sexual versus the wish to behave properly in public – is not conscious; the individual is not aware of it, but the strength of the conflict and the ensuing anxiety nevertheless influence his behaviour. Likewise, a fear of eating in public would be seen to arise out of the conflict to be greedy on the one hand and to behave in a proper manner on the other. The expressed fear of being sick is the imagined consequence of forbidden gluttony – the essence of greed, and the punishment of it. Fear of travelling would be seen as a wish to be carried away (by strong feelings) versus a fear of the social consequences were one to lose control of such feelings.

Analytic interpretations of this type may be valid for the specific subject of the analysis, but the big question remains to what extent such 'discoveries' can be extended into a general theory. There is always a danger in proceeding too uncritically from the specific to the general. Perhaps all that can be said is that such theories remind us that the anxiety and fear which the phobic patient experiences are very complicated and may arise from sources other than a simple fear of the object or situation. After all, these fears are recognized as irrational by the patient and are seen not to make sense in reality. The psychodynamic theory offers one explanation for this irrationality, by placing the origin of the anxiety in our inner, largely unconscious and private worlds.

(2) Behavioural explanations

Learning is a basic property of the brain which arises out of its inherent structure. The intermeshing of the thousands of branching nerve cells ensures that connections are made between events occurring in the brain over time. Learning is an intellectual process of making connections between otherwise disparate events: if two events occur in the brain in close temporal association, the brain 'learns' to link these two events together. A links with B, B links with C, and A links with C by way of its intermediary link with B. Learning consists of the erection of many interrelated chains of such linkages.

This learning process can be studied in laboratory conditions. A dog will naturally salivate if food is placed in front of it. This is a normal physiological response, and the food is called an unconditioned stimulus (UCS) for salivation. If, each time food is placed in front of the dog, a bell of a certain tone and pitch is rung immediately afterwards, the dog over time associates the bell with food and salivation, so that ultimately the dog will salivate if the bell is rung on its own. The bell has become a conditioned stimulus (CS) for salivation. If, thereafter, every so often food is placed before the dog at the same time as the bell and salivation, the salivation response is perpetuated or reinforced. Otherwise, the linkage between food, the bell and salivation weakens over time, and the conditioned stimulus is said to attenuate, or be extinguished. Anything which reduces a physiological drive (answers hunger, reduces anxiety, provides sexual release) will also reinforce a conditioned stimulus.

Food ——————→ salivation (UCS)
Food + bell ——————→ salivation
Bell ——————→ salivation (CS)

Bell (+ food) ——————→ salivation (reinforcement of CS)
Bell (+ no food) - - - - - - - - - - → less salivation (extinction of CS)

Bell (+ satisfaction of hunger)
——————→ salivation (drive reduction and reinforcement of CS)

Anxiety and fear are powerful drives and are involved in learning situations. Experimental animals will learn to associate originally neutral stimuli with fear (CS), and anything which reduces anxiety or fear will reinforce this particular conditioned response. Behavioural explanations of phobias are based on similar conditioned learning in human beings. Otherwise neutral situations become conditioned stimuli for a fear response (phobic dread), by the temporal association of these neutral stimuli with some anxiety-provoking event (the unconditioned stimulus). For example, someone is walking in the street; suddenly they feel anxious and panicky because they have just witnessed an accident. This natural and understandable anxiety response becomes attached to the otherwise neutral setting of the street. Because this person has the capacity to anticipate panic at some future date in the street, this reinforces the conditioned fear response. Anticipating fear in the mind is equivalent to experiencing fear in reality. Refusing to go into that street thereafter, to avoid possible panic, lowers the anxiety drive and again reinforces the conditioned stimulus of 'street equals fear response'. The phobia consists of the learned fear response, plus the avoidance behaviour. The phobia is established, and the irrational fear of the street is explained.

Such behavioural explanations are more credible the more the fear is aroused by a specific object or situation, such as heights, storms or aeroplanes. They seem less easy to apply to complex patterns of anxiety to many stimuli, as in agoraphobia. It can be argued that there is a central conditioned fear, which then generalizes to a variety of associated situations – fear of the street is central; fear of shops, crowds, traffic and so on are associated features which become linked into the central fear. Separation anxiety can also be understood in such terms. The original security which mother or both parents represented becomes linked with the home. Leaving home then evokes the same anxiety (conditioned response) as would be released by enforced separation as a child from the parents (unconditioned response). Returning home reduces the anxiety drive and thus reinforces the desire to remain in the home so as to avoid the separation anxiety and panic.

Just as the psychodynamic explanation is linked to a historical case, Little Hans, so the behavioural explanation is linked with a paper published by Watson and Rayner in 1920. Once more the subject is a little boy, in this case called Albert. Watson decided to test the theory of conditioned fear response in humans in the laboratory. Like many young children, Albert liked handling small furry white animals, in his case a white rabbit or white rat. He was not afraid. In the experiment, every time he picked up the animal, a metal bar was struck soundly behind his head, frightening him with the loud and unexpected noise. Gradually he transferred his fear of the noise to a fear of the animal. Furthermore, fear of the white animal generalized to anything which was white and of a similar texture. Watson had demonstrated a learned and conditioned fear response, together with generalization, in a human being. He also demonstrated the opposite: that the learned fear could be extinguished by the use of a counteracting stimulus – in Albert's case a sweet and warm reassurance every time he approached the feared animal, until he could pick it up again. He did so with caution, but there was no acute fear.

The behavioural explanation of phobias does not require any postulate such as the unconscious conflict inherent in the psychodynamic explanation, but requires only an intact nervous system, an initial anxiety-provoking stimulus and a susceptible subject within which the conditioning can occur. It might be asked, therefore, why more people are not prey to phobic anxiety. The answer lies in the relative balance of fear-inducing and fear-reducing factors in individuals, who will have a varying capacity for conditioned learning. Studies show that anxious, tense people are more prone to conditioned learning than those who are naturally more calm and relaxed in their attitudes to life. As an explanation it does satisfy the mystery of the irrational element of the fear, and the persistence of the phobia once established – a conditioned response, and reinforcement through avoidance.

(3) Ethological and social explanations

Animals naturally avoid potentially life-threatening situations and early on learn to recognize friend and foe. Anything which is different is possibly dangerous: young rabbits 'freeze' when the shadow of a hawk passes overhead; birds will mob one of their own kind which has been coloured with an artificial dye. Fear of animals and reptiles is common in man and in primates. Fear of snakes goes well beyond any real danger which the snake represents – the slow writhing movements, the hissing sound, the silent gliding across the floor and the stealthy approach all induce acute fear. Animals dislike being stared at and will not maintain eye-to-eye contact; likewise some people are afraid of, and believe in, the Evil Eye. This power is attributed to persons who are strange, different and therefore potentially dangerous – tinkers, gipsies and foreigners of all kinds are believed to be capable of bringing misfortune just by looking in a certain way. Fear and avoidance in all these examples serve to protect the individual and preserve the species – they have a biological survival value.

Studies show that cornered animals have a relatively limited way of dealing with threat: they can attack the aggressor, they can escape out of the situation as quickly as possible, or they can submit to the stronger animal and fend off attack by displaying a submission posture, which switches off the aggressor's drive to attack. It can be argued that humans have literally the same options in social encounters – attack, flight or submission – and also in their psychological defences against threat anxiety: attack through obsessional control, submission through neurotic passivity (hysterical or schizoid defences) and finally flight through phobic defences. In *obsessional defences* the individual seeks to control his environment in every particular detail, so that in effect nothing can be unknown, every contingency has been thought of and appropriate responses worked out. An overall sense of mastery neutralizes the anxiety of insecurity and doubt. In *hysterical or schizoid defences* the individual demonstrates extreme passivity towards the environment: he appears to be helpless and incapable of asserting himself in any way. He presents himself as the plaything of fate and apparently reconciled to any outcome; but only apparently so, because this is a defence designed to ward off fate and danger. In *phobic defences* the individual escapes from the immediate source of danger and arranges to avoid it at all costs in the future. There is a movement away from danger towards what is felt to be security.

All three defences can be seen in phobic disorders. The patient needs to feel in full control of himself and of his environment, and thus is doubly anxious when he feels he is losing control, as occurs in the common fear of losing consciousness, of fainting, or of committing some socially forbidden act. There is a retreat into safety, where the individual feels more in control of himself; elaborate precautions have to be taken to ward off approach to such danger in the future. In the face of repeated attacks of anxiety and panic, phobic patients feel totally helpless; there is nothing they can do about them; they will happen time and time again; the patients are defeated by their dilemma and largely give up trying to fight against it. Finally, there is a literal phobic flight away from the feared situation back to the place of safety – the home or another capable human being – and studied avoidance of that situation thereafter. These psychological and emotional defences in this context are to be understood less in their psychodynamic sense and more as survival strategies remaining from our evolutionary past. Modern society is not a jungle full of predatory animals but it is a location of growing social competition, threat and often violence. The threats are both physical to our persons and psychological to our well-being and self-confidence; our bodies are threatened but so also are our internal private worlds of mental symbols.

(4) Individual commonsense explanations

Many patients, in their escape from ambiguity and in their search for meaning, fall back on what can be called commonsense or obvious explanations for what they know to be irrational and mysterious behaviour. These explanations are a kind of whistling in the dark, because they do not really satisfy but bring about a sort of comfort for the time being. Patients examine their lives and find that they are under a lot of stress and strain; they think that this may have exhausted their coping mechanisms to such an extent that they are now having a nervous breakdown, of which the phobia is the major symptom. Others feel dissatisfied with their life-style: there seems so little pleasure and reward for effort; their roles at home or at work bring little satisfaction;

they do not like what they have, but equally do not know what they would like instead. They see the phobia as a result of this conflict or of boredom – a sign that things are not as they ought to be. In some there is a family history of a close relative who was similarly affected, so the phobia is seen as an inherited characteristic, something which runs in the family and therefore has just got to be put up with. Others torment themselves with a tyrannical self-judgement, seeing the phobia as a sign of personal weakness in the face of life's battles; they despise themselves and feel ashamed, trying to hide their defect from others. Some see it as a natural exaggeration of basic shyness or timidity, something which they have to learn to grow out of, if only they knew how. Because of the irrationality and mystery of it all, many give up trying to understand it, and see it as evidence that they are going out of their minds.

As with all commonsense explanations of life, there is more than a grain of truth in such suppositions, but as many questions are begged as are answered. These are only starting-points: the meaning and significance of a particular phobia in a particular person have to be sought for carefully. Sweeping generalizations are dangerous and misleading. In some the psychodynamic explanation will suffice; in others the behavioural approach makes better sense. The ethological explanation is more philosophic and speculative, but provides a background against which the other two models of explanation can be finally judged. Attempts are being made to reinterpret each model in terms of the others, thereby releasing new insights and new questions for further research.

To demonstrate the interdependence of these causal factors, certain questions can be asked in the evaluation of a particular phobia:

(a) Is there a family history of phobia – support for a genetic contribution to the illness and to a phobia-prone personality, as well as support for a family learning pattern, that is, a cultural and social contribution?
(b) Is there a true dread of an external situation rather than a more primary fear of leaving the home – support for a true phobic disorder rather than for separation anxiety?
(c) Is there a clear-cut initial incident of anxiety or panic based on events in reality which becomes the nucleus of a subsequent phobia – support for a behavioural learning theory causation?
(d) If (c) is not the case, is there evidence of an underlying psychological or emotional conflict which is being served by the phobia or

enacted through it – support for a psychodynamic symbolic causation?

(e) Is there marked and well-established avoidance behaviour – support for both a behavioural causation (drive reduction) and a psychodynamic causation (resolution of inner conflict)?

(f) Are there cultural and social factors which make the patient more likely to be phobic – support for the view that the phobia is an expression of the particular circumstances of the patient and the family, in cultural and social terms?

In all such evaluations it must be remembered that these causal factors are not mutually exclusive but do interact with each other. Whichever explanation is decided upon at the end of the day will be important in the patient's better understanding of why the illness has developed, and it will also suggest which method of treatment is most likely to be helpful for this particular patient and family.

CHAPTER 6
THE BIRTH AND GROWTH OF A PHOBIA

Irrespective of the various theories of how phobias come about, there seems to be a fairly constant pattern to the beginning and growth of the disorder. A phobia does not just appear out of the blue, but develops and grows over time. Many patients remember vividly the day on which they had their first panic attack, but closer questioning reveals that there are nearly always events which have gone before, to prepare the way, as it were, for the emergence of the full-blown phobia. We should not be surprised at this, because whether the origins of phobias are seen in unconscious conflicts or arise out of learned responses to stress, the phobia itself is a constellation of features which come to be associated together, and this association takes time to build up.

Studies of individual life histories by Brown and his colleagues at Bedford College, London, show that there are significant life events which render the individual more or less susceptible to stress and threat. These life events are nodal points in the chain of evolution of a particular biography. They occur at shifts from one stage of life to another, such as from adolescence to adulthood, from being a child of one's own parents to being a parent of one's own child and so on. Engagements, marriages, births, divorces and deaths all have similar effects; at such times of internal psychological change to external social change, we are for a time more vulnerable and deal less well with threat, anxiety, fear and danger. Thus, it can be predicted that external events occurring at such times will be more likely to start off a phobic process, which will be sustained and developed if the right circumstances prevail thereafter.

Although there is no specific 'pre-phobic' personality type, people will be more likely to develop a phobia the more they are anxiety-prone, sensitive to external and internal pressures and generally lacking in self-confidence. For some people the ground is prepared from birth onwards: they grow up to be more sensitive, anxious and insecure. They carry the potential to be afraid and experience panic, and want to avoid circumstances which they have come to realize evoke such feelings. Mention has already been made of Abe's experience in Japan and of Berg in England, of the connection between school phobia in childhood and the emergence of other phobias in adulthood in such predisposed persons. But this is not the whole story: many people who develop a phobia in adult life appear to be strong, self-reliant and not particularly anxious; they cope with life and its vicissitudes very well. Why do they develop a phobia? An answer might be that either, deep inside them, they have particular conflicts or susceptibilities not yet activated and thus not intrusive into behaviour, until provoked later, or else they meet an initiating event at one of the nodal points in their life story. Quite commonly patients say that their lives were entirely free of trouble until after they married, or a child was born, or a close relative died, or they were promoted to a new job. They will characteristically declare that these events did not upset them, nor are they the source of obvious strain, but each does represent a considerable shift in their public and private circumstances.

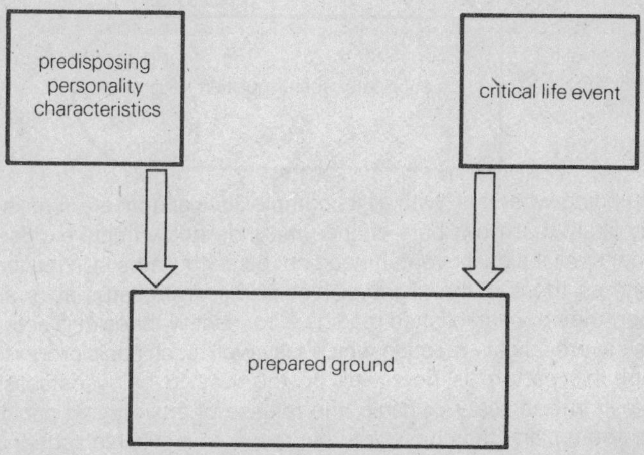

The stage is now set for what can be called the *signal event* – something which happens to evoke a normal anxiety response. This can be anything – witnessing a road accident, feeling unwell in the street, feeling faint in the supermarket because of the noise and heat, realizing one might be sick in a restaurant, finding evidence for what could be serious illness in oneself, being involved in a non-fatal accident, train crash or aeroplane failure. The anxiety experienced is perfectly normal and understandable. However, in the predisposed individual this event sets up currents and vortices of secondary anxiety – what if it happened again? how would I cope with it the next time? if it happens again, will I survive a second time? This rumination on what has happened generates a secondary anticipatory predisposition which compounds the first.

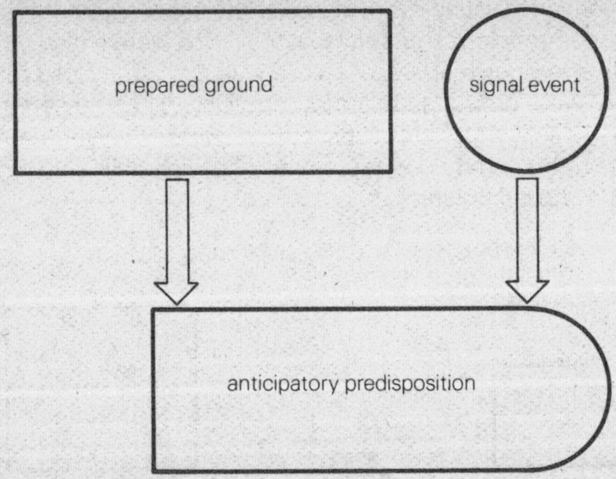

Life being what it is, with all its complexities and inherent risks, it is highly likely that from pure chance the individual will be exposed to another similar signal event. It need not be so frightening in reality, but as long as there is the slightest hint of discomfort, threat or actual danger, the now established readiness to react with alarm is activated into a severe anxiety reaction which may well reach panic proportions. The phobic pattern is now well on the way to being established: anticipation of anxiety or panic, the release of anxiety and panic in a given setting, and the conviction that this is an inevitable sequence of events in such a setting.

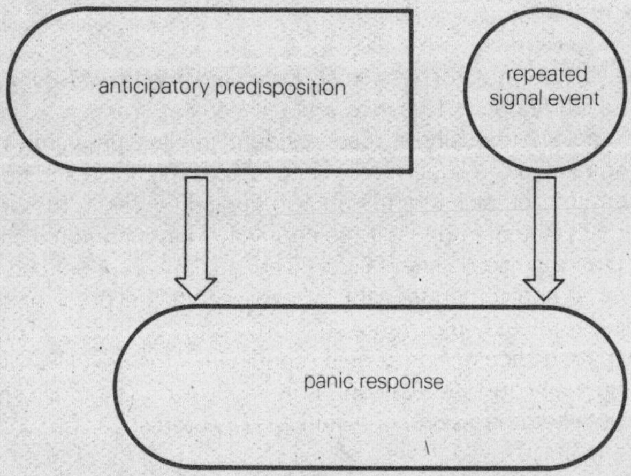

The experience of the panic itself, or even the anticipation of it happening, is so distressing and disturbing to most people that they will naturally try to avoid putting themselves into a situation where they believe, rightly or wrongly, that it will always happen. As a result they begin to develop complicated avoidance behaviour which serves to protect them from this risk.

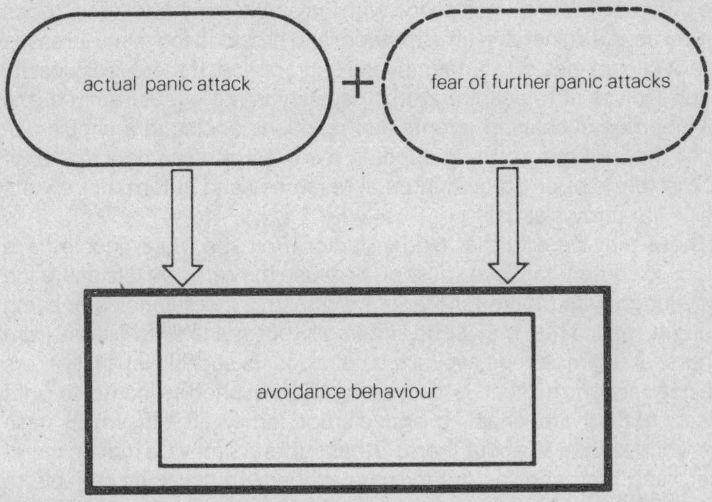

The phobia is now fully grown. The patients know that certain settings have released anxiety, fear and panic in them; they are convinced that this is an inevitable consequence of going into such settings, so they make sure that they avoid them at all costs, even though this avoidance may be inconvenient or embarrassing, or disrupt the pattern of family life.

For many patients suffering from a phobia, such a developmental explanation makes sense. For others the pattern of growth is less clear because the mind 'forgets' what it wants to forget, forgets what was painful, distressing or shaming. In such cases the phobia may appear to come out of the blue, unannounced and thus totally inexplicable. However, a careful study of the patient's history, especially if they are willing to try to remember antecedent events, will gradually reveal a similar build-up over time; the phobia, although distressing and inconvenient, is no longer a mystery, but something which can be understood and thus possibly brought under conscious control. It is not a sign of madness, or of personal moral weakness; it is a complex pattern of behaviour emerging out of given encounters and serving a specific purpose.

One last thought: since life is dangerous, and since we are all a bit anxious from time to time and accidents do happen, why do more people not develop phobias? Many people do have their own specific fears, but not full-blown phobic disorders. It is a matter of timing and the prepared ground; many cope with inevitable stress provided it does not come at a vulnerable time for them and provided too many stresses do not pile up, one on another, over a short period. If there is a capacity in the individual to adapt and that capacity is not over-stretched, the developmental chain of events and reactions ending in a phobic disorder may not get off the ground. In many ways it can be a matter of luck in terms of one's own internal resources and in terms of events which life throws at us.

There may be a further hidden factor. Perhaps more people have phobic disorders than we know of, because they are afraid to share the knowledge with others for fear of ridicule, misunderstanding or being thought mad. They may suffer internally but manage to hide it from others, or organize their avoidance behaviour in such a way that others do not recognize what is happening. Some phobias come to light because they are crippling and disrupt family life, in which case everyone knows all about them. Other sufferers may be more circumspect and their phobias more circumscribed, so that they are able to keep all knowledge of the disorder, and their private ways of dealing with it, secret. Only if these ways of coping begin to fail will others begin to suspect, and what has been kept private will then become public.

CHAPTER 7
THE MANAGEMENT AND TREATMENT OF PHOBIAS

The management of an illness means the overall care of the patient and involves both an understanding of the illness and a coming to terms with it, which may or may not include modification of the symptoms to make life more bearable. Treatment implies an attempt to eradicate the illness so that the patient may return to a previous level of satisfactory health and functioning. All illnesses are manageable, but not all are treatable. There is a subtle balance between the patient's wish to escape out of the constraints of the illness, and their capacity and willingness to cooperate with the therapist in eradicating the disorder. Some patients have more resolve, more determination, more support and less crippling disorders and thus have a good chance of recovery, whereas others are more overwhelmed by the illness and less endowed with resolve and the means by which to combat the condition. Therefore, in an overall management programme, there will be a sensitive balance between helping the patient come to terms and to live with the disorder, and helping them to fight a way out of the maze of pain and fearfulness.

Just as there are several theories of causation of phobic illnesses, so there are several treatment approaches based on an understanding of what has gone wrong and how it might therefore be put right. These treatment approaches fall under three main headings: physical treatments, psychoanalytic treatments and behaviour therapy treatments. Each takes the patient, caught up in the inevitability of a phobic fear response with the associated avoidance behaviour, and tries to break the total behaviour pattern to allow a degree of new learning and re-training to take place. Each seeks to enable the patient to break out of the bonds of the illness and re-discover a previous level of better functioning over time.

An *overall management programme*, for whatever type of phobic disorder is present, should consist of the following steps:

(a) exploration and diagnosis
(b) explanation and understanding
(c) modification of the symptoms
(d) eradication through new learning and re-training
(e) review and reinforcement of improvement
(f) long-term follow-up of the outcome

An essential first step is careful and detailed investigation of the patient's history to ensure that the preliminary diagnosis is correct. The word 'phobia' is used so frequently nowadays that certain disorders are too loosely described as phobic when they may well be a totally different condition requiring a totally different approach. In particular, *primary phobic disorders* must be distinguished from *secondary phobic symptoms*, the treatment of which is the treatment of the underlying causal illness. Primary phobias in turn must be distinguished from separation anxiety disorders, acute anxiety states, obsessional compulsive states, pan-phobic reactions and a generalized loss of confidence, for whatever reason, in insecure, vulnerable people who just cannot cope with life and its many pressures.

Exploration of the pattern of the disorder – how it began, how it grew and developed, how the symptoms are released, how the patient has learned various ways of coping with them – allows an understanding of the overall behaviour pattern to be grasped; whether the disorder is seen to arise out of inner conflict or from learned avoidance behaviour, it is no longer a mystery, often believed to be early evidence of insanity, but an understandable sequence of events, leading to an established pattern of behaviour. Understanding what is happening is often the first step to doing something about it.

All patients need encouragement to have the strength to face the illness, and to begin to fight against it on the long road back to recovery. Fear and anxiety rapidly destroy resolve, and so anything which helps the patient to feel more comfortable releases energy to be used in fighting the illness. Furthermore, feeling better allows many people to have a first hope that perhaps, after all, they may be able to begin to escape out of the net in which they find themselves.

Now begins the hard part – the conscious and deliberate attempt to learn new ways of dealing with the primary cause, whether it derives from inner conflict or from maladaptive learning. This means re-training responses at both a conscious and an unconscious level. It means opening oneself up to risk, taking chances, lowering habitual defences to allow new patterns to evolve. It means facing and staying rather than turning and fleeing. It means controlling the disorder rather than letting it do the controlling.

New learning comes in stages, and slipping back often occurs as well as striding forwards: there are both snakes and ladders in the game of recovery. Disappointment and disillusionment are understandable and have to be faced as well as the illness itself. This requires constant encouragement from others, and continuous redefining of the management programme. All gains have to be consolidated; all failures evaluated, but above all kept in perspective: a temporary slipping back does not necessarily mean 'going back to square one'. Re-education and re-learning are continuous and forward-looking processes. There is no room for looking back save to identify mistakes so that they are less likely to happen again.

Finally, it is important to take a long perspective look at what has been achieved, to ensure that the new learning has been maintained and that old habits of compromise and avoidance are not creeping back. It is so easy to give up before the new hard-won learning has reached a point of stabilization, in which the old habitual behaviour has been removed and the new way of dealing with things has itself in turn become habitual.

(1) Physical treatment approach

Physical treatments aim to improve the patient's psychological and emotional state by mechanical means such as by drugs, electrical treatment (ECT) and psycho-surgery (leucotomy). Physical treatments are designed to blank out existing patterns of behaviour and response, in order to allow the individual to return to his previous level of reasonable function, or to clear the way for new adaptive learning to take place.

Drug therapy. Drugs are used in the first instance by many doctors because they are relatively cheap, relatively effective and available for use while the patient continues to live at home. In phobias, because of the excessive anxiety, *tranquillizers* of all kinds are the drugs of first choice. A tranquillizer ideally calms the patient without producing the drowsiness which is a drawback in the use of sedatives by day. At the present time there are some thirty-six tranquillizers available on prescription in the UK, of which Librium (chlordiazepoxide) and Valium (diazepam) are the best known and have been available for a long time. There is a new generation of tranquillizers now on the market, such as Frisium (clobazam), Nobrium (medazepam) and Serenid–D (oxazepam). All work in similar ways – shielding the patient from the assaults of external stress and diminishing the internal physiological response to that stress. Such drugs are psycho-active, that is they alter consciousness, or at least the conscious response to stress. Other drugs, such as Inderal (propranolol), a ß blocking agent, are less psycho-active and work by dampening down the peripheral effects of anxiety – sweating, trembling, palpitations and so on. Bernadt and his colleagues in London in 1980 reported the effect of a ß blocker (Tolanol) compared to Valium (diazepam) and a placebo (chemically inert substance) on twenty-two female subjects suffering from spider or snake phobias. While the

Tolanol controlled the palpitations of the panic attacks, it had little effect on how the subject felt about the phobic object or on how she behaved in its presence. Valium did not alter the palpitations, but the subject's behaviour in the presence of the phobic object improved. Other studies confirm that ß blockers are best used in short-term conditions of disabling anxiety, such as examination nerves or stage fright, rather than in the prolonged anxiety of phobic states.

All tranquillizers, while relatively safe in the short term, carry the danger of habituation and dependence in the long term – the patient has to take more and more for a given effect, coming to rely on the drug, so that when it is discontinued a variety of unpleasant withdrawal effects are experienced. This does not always happen, but there is a decided risk in some dependent personalities. Such drugs should only be taken under medical advice, and then only for a relatively short period, to begin a treatment programme or to get over particularly bad patches. Prolonged use, though it may seem an attractive idea at first, will ultimately be regretted. *Sedatives*, such as Dalmane (flurazepam), Euhypnos (temazepam) and Mogadon (nitrazepam), can also be of use for a time, to ensure a period of refreshing sleep ('sleep which knits up the ravell'd sleeve of care'). Otherwise, there is the same danger of habituation and dependency.

Interest has turned to the use of *antidepressants* in the treatment of primary phobias. Secondary phobic symptoms, released by an underlying depression, could be expected to respond logically to the treatment of the causal depression, but it is not fully known why primary phobias, without any depression, should improve on the use of a tricyclic antidepressant such as Anafranil (clomipramine), or of a monoamine oxidase inhibitor such as Nardil (phenelzine). In 1975, Tyrer reported on the use of Nardil (phenelzine) in the treatment of twenty-eight patients with agoraphobia and various social phobias. He showed that Nardil was comparable in effect to other treatments in these disorders and acted mainly by suppressing symptoms rather than altering the fundamental condition. With such drugs there is a need to be careful of possible interactions between these and other medicines or certain foodstuffs. As with tranquillizers, there is a real danger of dependency developing in long-term use. Mountjoy, in a study in 1977, demonstrated that Nardil could help in phobic states where there had been no previous response to tranquillizers such as Librium or Valium. The Nardil could be used on its own or combined with a tranquillizer for added effect. Then it was found that Anafranil (clomipramine) was effective in obsessional and phobic states. A technique of giving

Anafranil by intravenous drip was popular for a time, but most workers feel that this is not necessary provided the patient is able to take the drug by mouth and is absorbing it adequately from the alimentary canal. Antidepressant drugs have more marked side-effects than tranquillizers, which can upset patients, but these are often most marked in the early use of the drug and become less obvious when the dose is increased. Anafranil causes mainly a dry mouth and some constipation; there can also be slight blurring of vision and over-sedation in some people. At least the side-effects show that the drug is getting into the body system. With Anafranil, unlike Nardil, there is no need for caution with foodstuffs, except, as with all psycho-active drugs, alcohol.

Drugs can therefore be a help in the short term, by allowing patients to begin to feel better, which in turn gives hope and encouragement to go on to other treatments which influence the underlying disorder in the long term. A patient with a phobia can either have a tranquillizer such as Librium or Valium by day, with a sedative such as Dalmane at night, or try Anafranil as the drug of choice by day. Tranquillizers act more quickly than antidepressants, which should be taken for at least three weeks before being abandoned as useless. Any course of such drugs, singly or in combination, should be continued for at least six weeks to give the drugs a chance to act, and thereafter be reviewed every three months to prevent long-term dependency or habituation. This is less likely to develop if the drugs are kept to the minimum effective dose and the body given a rest from them from time to time. This allows an effective drug schedule to be kept in use over an extended period.

Electrical treatment (ECT) has no place in the treatment of primary phobias, but may be indicated in severe depressive illnesses, in which there can occasionally be phobic symptoms. Here, the electrical treatment is directed to the depressive illness and not to the phobic symptoms themselves.

Psycho-surgery (leucotomy) remains a contentious issue in modern psychiatry and is used very rarely indeed, because the need for the operation has been superseded by the development of more effective and more acceptable treatments. Psycho-surgery aims at interrupting nerve pathways believed to be involved in certain patterns of maladaptive behaviour, and can bring relief when there is unbearable tension in the patient which has failed to respond to other corrective measures. Marks and his colleagues at the Maudsley Hospital, London, reported in 1966 a retrospective study of leucotomies performed for a variety of reasons and identified twenty-two patients in which a modified operation had been carried out for anxiety and severe agoraphobia. They compared the operated group with matched controls for a five-year period after treatment. They showed that the leucotomy patients did significantly better than the controls for improvement in the phobias and anxiety; the anxiety showed maximum improvement within three months of the operation, whereas the phobias continued to show improvement after the first year. The outcome was less good in the case of a shy anxious personality with marked depression before the operation. They felt at the time that, in long-standing cases of agoraphobia, severe in quality and associated with marked anxiety, which had not responded satisfactorily to other treatments, modified leucotomy should be considered. The up-to-date view would be the same, but recognizing that the need for such operations is thankfully very rare.

(2) Psychoanalytic treatments approach

The psychoanalytic method is a means of contacting and identifying those mental processes which are not immediately conscious and making them available for introspection. Work with phobias is directed towards a search for meaning by identifying those internal events – memories, conflicts and ideals – which may lie behind the formation of the phobia, itself a way of dealing with tension, stress and inner distress. The psychoanalytic method may not be able to say why a phobia emerges rather than a depression or a non-phobic anxiety state, but it can often show why the phobia crystallizes around a particular situation and emerges as a particular social fear, or a constellation of related fears, as in agoraphobia. An examination of the symbolic content of the phobic behaviour may, by a process of decoding, give vital information about how this particular phobia has come about in this particular person's life. The psychoanalytic method can be used in various ways.

Classical psychoanalysis. This is very expensive and time-consuming, and almost inevitably, as the phobia is examined and understood, will reveal otherwise unexpected problems at a deeper level, like a series of self-containing Russian dolls. As a classical method it cannot be made available to the large number of people suffering from phobias, and at the same time it is an inappropriate way of dealing with a problem which is relatively accessible in most patients. Full analysis of the early cases, such as Little Hans, did, however, open doors to a deeper understanding of what otherwise at that time was inexplicable.

Analytic psychotherapy. This is derived from classical analytic theory and can be used in selective ways to focus on parts of a given patient's drama. It can be directed towards the examination of the phobic defence and how it does or does not protect the individual from his inner conflicts and stresses. It can be used to help to develop insight into the meaning of the phobia for that person in his overall life history, and need not take a very long time if therapist and patient focus on the phobia and do not allow themselves to be distracted into byways, no matter how interesting and intriguing.

Dynamic psychotherapy. This can be made available to a greater number of people as it does not require the same depth of penetration, and various techniques have been evolved which can be taught to suitable therapists without the full rigours of a personal analysis. Dynamic psychotherapy focuses upon the emotional and psychological processes at work inside the patient – his ways of identifying and solving problems, his insights and personal strategies for coping, his defence mechanisms and so on. The personality structure is the field within which these various dynamic processes have to be identified and scrutinized. Some psychotherapies remain with the present of the individual (here and now techniques). This transactional analysis examines the various ploys and 'games' people play to cope with the pressures of life in their everyday dramas of existence. Others relate present to past (there and then techniques), showing how old patterns of coping are repeated time and again, without necessarily being relevant to the current situation. Gestalt psychotherapy shows how the patients can make use of symptoms and disabilities to express certain truths about themselves and how they wish to be seen by others. The total pattern can be understood only by relating all the parts to a continuous background of the personal evolution of that particular patient.

All such psychoanalytically derived treatments can be given only by those who have been properly trained to do so and who themselves continue to be supervised in their work by more experienced colleagues. As a general method of treatment it has its limits and can help only a relatively few patients. The patient is either seen *individually* by one therapist or joins a *group* of similar patients, with one or more therapists. In 1977, Teasdale and his colleagues, from Oxford, reviewed the overall effectiveness of group exposure in a cohesive group for eighteen patients suffering from agoraphobia. There were three therapists and one in training. The method consisted of going out to face the situation which the patients feared, and then returning to discuss in the group how they felt and coped with what had happened. Although this method was not shown to be more effective than individual methods, it used the therapists' time more economically. Group therapy allows social-interaction processes to be examined and utilized in both the understanding and the management of phobias, which are very much public and social disorders. *Family therapy* is a natural progression from individual to group (strangers) to group (relatives). Phobias affect not only the patient but the whole family, who may be involved in maintaining the disorder and who all therefore can help in the eradication of this particular form of family behaviour.

Whatever psychoanalytic or psychodynamic method is used, the treatment programme can focus on the following:

(a) Possible hidden conflicts and motives.
(b) Reasons for the timing of onset of the phobia – why does it emerge at this stage of the patient's life?
(c) Resistances in the patient which may be maintaining the illness and, despite professed wishes to be better, keep the patient locked in an avoidance pattern.
(d) Reasons for the content of the phobia – why a social phobia rather than agoraphobia, and why a fear of vomiting rather than a fear of animals?
(e) The overall meaning of the illness in the patient's life history, the reassurance that comes through understanding, and the relief through mastery of ambiguity and self-doubt.

(3) Behaviour therapy approach

Behaviour therapy is based on learning theory, which holds that all behaviour, no matter how complex, is made up of a series of learned responses organized into a hierarchy. Illnesses such as phobias are seen as maladaptive, unsuitable learned responses which can therefore be corrected by unlearning the old habit and re-learning a new one, adaptive and more appropriate to the situation. The re-training takes place in full consciousness and requires the total and active cooperation of the patient, who is taught a personal training schedule. As with psychodynamic methods, there are various behaviour therapy treatments:

Relaxation methods. Anxiety is the result of sympathetic activity in the autonomic nervous system; anything which activates the opposite component, the parasympathetic, will neutralize anxiety. Active relaxation increases parasympathetic activity. Many people believe that relaxation is a natural and automatic behaviour, but nervous and tense people have forgotten how to relax and have to be taught a lost skill. Active relaxation sounds like a contradiction in terms, but it is possible to learn how to induce a relaxed state of mind and body. The mind gains active control over the body and, shutting out all distractions, wills each part of the body in turn to feel pleasantly comfortable and free from tension. Slow deep breathing further increases the overall relaxation, and the mind finally can focus on a mental picture of peace and tranquillity. There are a number of *methods of relaxation*, but they are all variations of a basic technique which can be taught to most people. Some, however, become tense just at the very thought of relaxing, because to them it is a kind of letting-go, an abandonment of control, the very thing they are most afraid of. Such individuals can be helped either by a *hypnotic technique*, or by a method developed by Friedman at St Bartholomew's Hospital, London, which he introduced in 1966. He uses a quick-acting sedative – methohexitone – by intravenous injection. This allows the patient to relax without losing consciousness. In 1971, Friedman reported on a series of 124 patients, with a mixture of agoraphobias, social phobias and mono-symptomatic fears, treated by this method. Each session lasted about fifteen minutes and was repeated some twelve times. While relaxed under the drug, the patient was encouraged to imagine himself in the situation he was most afraid of. He followed up these patients from six months to five years and showed that 38 per cent remained symptom-free, 51 per cent had definitely improved and only 11 per cent had shown no improvement at all. Relaxation by itself helps people to feel better, but in addition is the first step towards the next technique.

Desensitization requires the patient to associate being relaxed with a progressive build-up to full exposure to the feared situation. This association can be done in reality or in imagination. The latter is more convenient, and perhaps easier to start with. Imagination is quite appropriate to phobias constructed from anticipatory anxiety in the mind of the sufferer – just as his imagination has constructed terrors, so this same imagination can be put to work in banishing these self-erected terrors, replacing them with calmness and self-confidence. Some people have poor 'visual' imaginations, preferring to think in abstract terms: such patients can be taught to be more 'visual' by the use of hypnotic suggestion. For training in imagination to be really effective the patient must use every means at his disposal to create the effect of actually being in the feared situation – sight, hearing, smell, and touch and taste if appropriate. Mathews and colleagues in Oxford reported in 1976 the treatment of thirty-six women with agoraphobia, using both imagination and exposure to reality. The patients were followed up after sixteen sessions of each and again at six months thereafter, and no significant difference in the result was found. All the patients had to be encouraged to persist in their practice sessions and not to give up too soon. Training in imagination may prepare some people to face the real thing, but it failed to do so in this series. Imagination may not be 'real' enough, or reality too overwhelming, for learning to be carried over from imagination to real exposure.

Whether use is made of imagination or reality, a *desensitization hierarchy* is constructed by breaking down a complex behaviour pattern, such as going shopping, into a logical sequence of steps, starting from the conscious decision made at home to go shopping, then moving through getting ready, leaving the house, catching public transport (if appropriate), to arriving at the door of the shop before plunging into the crowds. In a training session the patient is encouraged to take a step at a time, using relaxation methods to induce a feeling of perfect calm and competence while doing so. If one step is too distressing, the patient is instructed to go back a few steps and take plenty of time, letting relaxation neutralize the pre-existing fear response. Having begun in imagination, the patient can now repeat the process in reality, taking time out to sit on a bench or look in a shop window while using the relaxation method to neutralize any excess anxiety. There is no hurry: better to take time to build up confidence slowly than rushing for an effect which can just as easily be lost. Each success encourages a move on to the next step. Watson and his colleagues in London in 1971 showed with ten adult patients suffering from long-standing specific phobias that prolonged exposure to the feared situation, either in imagination or in reality, was an effective therapeutic agent. They gave their patients two or three sessions, each lasting four to five hours. The patients had to remain in the feared situation – it was felt that avoidance was the factor perpetuating the phobic pattern.

Flooding is a technique related to prolonged exposure. The patient is encouraged to go right into the feared situation and to remain there without avoidance. This results in a massive stimulation of anxiety and panic. The patient discovers that, although distressed and desperate to escape, his heart does not stop, his breathing, though laboured, does not stop, and he does not faint or do whatever he feared he might. He has survived the worst. Over time, the physiological basis of the released anxiety and panic becomes exhausted, so that the patient is now unable to feel anxious or panic-stricken in the feared situation. In London in 1971, Marks and his colleagues showed that flooding was more effective than desensitization but was less acceptable to patients and therapists. They felt that flooding worked by blocking conditioned avoidance, reducing the fear by abreaction (letting out the feelings), experiencing survival which is usually not put to the test, and offering a challenge to the patient. Flooding is, however, dramatic and not all patients are willing to take part in such treatment, and, even if they are, they have to be accompanied by a therapist, not only to monitor progress but to ensure that the patient doesn't go away.

Modelling involves the therapist going with the patient into the feared situation and through a desensitization procedure. The presence of the therapist is encouraging and allows errors in the programme to be corrected at the crucial time. The therapist actively shapes the patient's performance; for example, the therapist waits outside a shop while the patient is sent inside for a particular purchase; the patient comes out and reports to the therapist, who checks for any errors in response and sends the patient back inside once more. Ultimately, the patients are encouraged to go through the whole pattern of behaviour from beginning to end all by themselves – they must learn to face their fears on their own, relying on their own resources: taking someone with them is a prop, and dependency on another person is built into the new behaviour pattern. Modelling is a good method with shy, anxious and insecure patients, as well as with those who do not learn the techniques correctly and thus require to be shown how to behave in the situation they fear.

Self-assertion training gives shy, anxious and insecure patients permission and encouragement to stand up for themselves, and to take the risk of being more outgoing and self-assertive. Such patients are often afraid of how others will respond to them if they try to be more assertive, anticipating disapproval and rejection. Phobic avoidance may result as a defensive response. Such patients can be taught how to be assertive and relaxed at the same time. Again, this appears to be a contradiction in terms, and requires special training if the patient is to be able to face up to the world, meet challenges half way, and stay and face rather than to turn and run. In Oxford in 1979, Phyllis Shaw used desensitization, flooding and self-assertive social skills training with thirty patients with social phobias. Each method was used over ten sessions and the results compared. She showed that each method was effective in reducing subjectively experienced fears; however, flooding was not acceptable to several patients, and self-assertive social skills training was very expensive of the therapist's time. She concluded that desensitization techniques were probably the most cost-effective method and the most acceptable to patients.

Running therapy belongs to a group of serious treatments for phobias which have appeared in the medical journals and which at first sight seem quite fanciful. They are based, however, on the sound behavioural theory that anything which diminishes or abolishes anxiety in the presence of the phobic stimulus will extinguish the phobic response. If a patient goes into a phobic situation and holds his breath as long as possible, the relief which comes from being able to breathe again will neutralize the phobic anxiety if the procedure is repeated often enough. Likewise, if a patient deliberately runs himself almost to the point of exhaustion and then goes into the phobic situation, the relief from resting, together with a body physiology in a state of some stress, means that the phobic anxiety will once more not be felt. Orwin, in Birmingham in 1974, reviewed a number of possible techniques which activate autonomic parasympathetic tone to counter anxiety or panic – eating, laughter, respiratory relief (breath holding) and vigorous physical exertion. He reported the successful treatment of a young woman with a phobia toward high-level lavatory cisterns, using the method of running close to the limit of tolerance, before sitting down beneath an example of her phobic object. An almost life-long phobia was removed following five short training sessions; at a five-month follow-up, she had maintained her improvement. Such an approach is probably best with simple mono-symptomatic phobias and, although apparently economic of patient and therapist time, would not be easy to apply to complex phobias in a social setting, especially if the patient had a need to remain inconspicuous.

Thought-stopping can be used with phobias of internal, as opposed to external, origin. Some patients ruminate on unpleasant thoughts, fearing that they have some dread disease or that they will behave in such a way as to put others at risk through their careless actions. Unpleasant guilt and anxiety-inducing thoughts plague the individual and they cannot get rid of them, much as they would like to, as if from an external phobic situation. In 1971, Kumar and Wilkinson, from Derby, described a method of thought-stopping in which patients with internal obsessional phobias are taught relaxation techniques. They are asked to describe in detail a typical sequence of phobic ruminations, and then on a shouted command from the therapist they must stop and switch on to thoughts of a pleasant, relaxed, pleasure-giving scene which each has chosen. Such training teaches the patient both to stop the apparently uncontrollable thought sequence and also to neutralize the associated anxiety with pleasurable visual and auditory imagery.

Just as psychotherapy can be given on an individual or group basis, so can these various behaviour therapies. The experience of the *group treatment* of weight problems by behavioural means (Weight Watchers) emphasizes the value of group support, and also of group competition – to be the first to reach a target, to be the first to get the biggest result and so on. Group work takes less of the therapist's time and, in this context, Marks at the Maudsley Hospital, London, has pioneered the training of 'nurse therapists', who can use behavioural techniques to teach phobic patients methods of relaxation and desensitization and accompany them in modelling and flooding.

There has been a sterile debate on whether psychotherapy or behaviour therapy is 'best' for phobias. The psychotherapy school has accused the behaviouralists of treating only symptoms and not the underlying disorder, warning them that symptom substitution would occur (exchange of one symptom for another). The behavioural school has accused the psychotherapists of a needlessly mystical and unscientific approach to what is an essentially easily understood process, challenging the psychotherapists to 'prove' that psychotherapy works in a scientific sense, and countering that symptom substitution does not occur in practice. The debate is essentially futile because different patients have different problems and will respond to different methods. In 1967, Gelder with his colleagues in Oxford set up a prospective trial of desensitization and two forms of psychotherapy in phobic out-patients. Sixteen patients received desensitization, sixteen group psychotherapy and ten individual psychotherapy. Each treatment group contained agoraphobics as well as some with social phobias. Desensitization lasted on average for nine months, individual psychotherapy for one year and group psychotherapy for eighteen months. After six months of treatment symptoms had improved faster with desensitization than with psychotherapy, but by one year after treatment had begun, the psychotherapy patients had caught up, and these two groups went on improving slowly. A less good response, whatever method was used, was obtained with agoraphobic patients and in those who were older and obsessional. In particular, symptom substitution did not occur. Gelder concluded that all the treatment methods helped the patients and that there is not one preferred method. The one which commends itself to particular patients and to particular therapists should be employed.

(4) A combined approach

Although for convenience and simplicity it is easier to describe these various treatments separately, they are best used in combination as part of an overall management programme. In 1974 Snaith, from Wakefield, described his combined approach, which is based on preliminary explanation of what is to happen, the use of hypnosis to induce relaxation and vivid visual imagery for desensitization, and finally autogenic training – a means of self-induced relaxation through a set of prescribed exercises. The patient uses the autogenic training in preparation at home and can then employ it in reality. Like Gelder, Snaith believes that there is no set way of doing things, and that the patient and doctor or therapist have to work out together what is the best approach to each particular problem, taking into account the individual patient's resources and capabilities. Whatever is done must make sense to the patient if he is to cooperate.

A *comprehensive management programme* for any phobic disorder can be built up from the following elements, allowing for modification to suit individual cases:

(a) A detailed case-history taking in order to establish the diagnosis of a true phobic disorder.
(b) A simple explanation of the nature of phobic disorders, and why they persist despite the patient's wish to be better.
(c) An attempt to understand the patient's anxieties in terms of current conflicts and the influence of past events in the history.
(d) The preliminary use of a tranquillizer or related drug by day, and possibly a hypnotic at night, in cases of very anxious and insecure patients who need some help to get started and hope that they can begin to feel better.
(e) A simple explanation of the treatment approach to be used and the part the patient will be expected to play in it.

(f) A simple system of relaxation exercises which the patient will practise at home.
(g) The choice of a calm scene personal to the patient and to be used in desensitization later.
(h) The definition of the phobic stimulus and the circumstances for the patient in which it is likely to operate.
(i) The construction of a desensitization hierarchy to be used in training sessions at home, starting in imagination and then going out into the real situation when the patient feels able to do so.
(j) Regular follow-up sessions to check the relaxation and desensitization techniques and to record progress.
(k) A switch to other techniques such as modelling or flooding if the patient cannot use relaxation and desensitization, and possible use of group treatment for added encouragement and support.

It can be helpful for some patients to keep a progress diary in which they record what they have been able to do and a score which they give themselves for effort and achievement. This allows them to take responsibility for what is happening and keeps the progress in perspective, so that they are less likely to be upset by the occasional relapse.

A *good response* to such a management programme will be obtained only if the patient wants to give up the phobic avoidance behaviour and is prepared to cooperate actively with the therapist. The family likewise must be in tune with the general intent of therapy and not do anything which could detract from its purpose. The patient must be prepared to face the fear and not run away from it. This means ultimately going alone into the situation which is feared in order to learn to rely on internal resources. The use of drugs, helpful in the beginning, must be medically reviewed and then cautiously reduced and withdrawn at some stage of the treatment programme so that once more the patient is able to face the phobic stimulus drawing upon personal resources. Above all, the patient must be prepared to spend time actively pursuing the relaxation and desensitization exercises, whether in imagination or in reality.

A *less good response* is to be expected where an incorrect diagnosis has been made and the condition too loosely called a primary phobic disorder, particularly in very insecure and generally anxious patients who often find the treatment more threatening than their basic condition. Some patients and families learn to 'adapt' around the phobia, and may have little to gain in going back to the pre-phobic organization of the family group. Others may be using the phobia for secondary gain and thus may not be prepared to give up its advantages despite the inconveniences of the condition. Some patients are unwilling or unable to cooperate actively with the therapist and, whatever method is used, in their passivity are hoping for a 'magical' cure, independent of their own effort and involvement in the treatment programme.

(5) Self-help and treatment at home

Because of the natural tendency for patients and relatives to rely on the skill and help given to them by various therapists, and the danger of a passive dependency developing which can work against the patient discovering for himself how to combat and face his fears using his own resources, increasing emphasis is being put on self-help groups and patient-directed training programmes.

Mathews and colleagues in Oxford reported in 1977 a home-based treatment programme for agoraphobia, to be managed by the patient in the home from the very beginning. The patient's married partner was actively involved in the planning and encouragement of the training sessions, and both patient and spouse were asked to take overall responsibility for organizing the treatment programme themselves. In order that they should know in detail what to do and what to expect, treatment manuals were devised explaining how the treatment would work, together with a simple step-by-step system for exercises and practice sessions. Such an approach can be used only where the marital and social adjustment of husband and wife is good, but when used it does diminish the risk of therapist dependence and allows the patient to attribute all improvement to personal effort, thus increasing self-confidence and competence.

Dr Claire Weekes, an Australian physician, has specialized in helping people with agoraphobia. She places great emphasis on a simple and practical approach to treatment. In her method, a combination of psychotherapy and behaviour therapy, she makes use of specially written books (*Self-Help for Your Nerves*, Angus and Robertson, 1962, and *Peace from Nervous Suffering*, Angus and Robertson, 1972) and tape recordings. Her system is based on:

(a) An attitude to the patient's trouble which is simple, practical and direct.
(b) Helping the patient to understand the meaning of the phobia.
(c) Constant repetition of advice and support through the medium of her books and tape recordings.
(d) Simple, clear-cut instructions based on four principles:

facing – that is acknowledging the nature of the problem and the distress that it causes, and not denying it.
accepting – that is living with the problem, accepting that it exists and not fighting against its existence.
floating – that is going along with the panicky feelings, not resisting them, but learning to continue to survive in their presence.
letting time pass – that is relaxing with the problem, going along with it and not fighting it against a time limit. She teaches that approaching the problem slowly and consistently will in the end bring better results.

Dr Weekes reminds her patients that relapses will happen from time to time and that this is understandable and inevitable. She emphasizes the importance of accepting the setback, not fighting it, and certainly not seeing it as a disaster or a reason for 'going back to square one'. Her method therefore combines aspects of psychodynamic understanding, relaxation and desensitization over time.

Apart from the medical advice and help that all patients require, there are other more personal and social aspects of care that they find that they can best give each other. Based on the model of Alcoholics Anonymous for people with drinking problems, a number of *self-help groups* for people with phobic problems have been set up, largely through the efforts of a particular patient or relative. The principle of mutual help is summed up in the slogan 'We alone can do it, but we can't do it alone'. Such self-help groups focus on competence rather than illness. They stress the need for people to join together to encourage each other to succeed, by demonstrating what they have been able to do rather than what they have failed to do. A medical approach must by its nature focus on the illness and the degree of disability, whereas self-help used as a supplement to professional help focuses on competitive and mutually supportive achievement. To rely totally upon a professional for help is to declare one's total dependence upon that person; to acknowledge that self-help is possible is to acknowledge that one is not totally powerless but can and must make a substantial contribution to the effort to escape from the disorder and its disabling effects.

There are a number of organizations that can be approached (see Some Useful Addresses, p. 101). If the phobic sufferer is desperate and feeling despondent, dejected or suicidal, the local branch of the *Samaritans* will offer friendship and a listening ear. The telephone numbers of

Samaritan branches are in local telephone directories. In 1965, a lady, herself a sufferer from agoraphobia, set up a correspondence information service which has now grown into *The Open Door Association*. There is also *The Phobics Society* and *The Phobic Trust*. The National Association for Mental Heath (*MIND*) has an information officer and a well-stocked book room with books and articles for those who wish to read more about all kinds of psychological and emotional disorders. MIND has branch offices in Gateshead, Preston, Sheffield, Leeds and Cardiff, whose addresses and telephone numbers can be obtained from the London office.

The management of phobias can now be seen to be complicated, like a map with many roads running to one destination. Which road a particular patient will have to travel to reach success will depend on a number of factors – the type of the phobia, its particular causes, the length of the illness, the availability of various technical and specialist services. Whatever route is taken, the road is a hard one, but the reward is not only a loss of phobic anxiety but a general improvement in self-confidence which comes from the patient's personal effort.

CHAPTER 8
OUTCOME STUDIES

For a patient prognosis is as important as diagnosis. The patient wants to know not only what is wrong but also what the outcome will be. What will happen to a given patient once a diagnosis has been made will depend both on the natural history of the disorder and on whether it is treated or not. Some disorders are by their nature fatal, and after a brief interlude the patient will die; other disorders are not fatal but will lead to the patient's steady deterioration into a state of increasing incapacity; other disorders come and go, with periods of disability followed by periods of improvement; and other disorders occur once in a patient's life and get better never to recur again. Phobias, by their nature, are not fatal, but they can become chronic and lead to progressive disablement, the patient becoming a virtual prisoner in the home (the housebound housewife). Phobias can also be recurrent, with episodes of relative freedom from excessive anxiety; and they can occur once in a lifetime and never again.

It is difficult to establish the natural history of a disorder such as a phobia because so many people are aware of the condition and come to the medical profession for treatment. Thus most of the outcome studies in phobias are based on follow-up assessment of cohorts of patients who have been treated once upon a time. Because of the great frequency of phobic fears in childhood, and the condition known as school phobia or school refusal, studies have been made of the frequency with which children who start off with childhood phobic fears go on to a school phobia and then to a phobic illness in adult life. Some of these studies have already been mentioned. The Japanese study of Abe from Osaka showed that, in a series of 242 mothers, 35 per cent of those who had marked childhood fears of thunder, animals or injections were still suffering from them in adult life. Berg's study in 1976 showed that those mothers who themselves had had school phobia had a greater tendency to have children who themselves would suffer from that condition, and that those mothers had an earlier onset of agoraphobia than mothers without school phobia. He also followed up, for seven years, 125 adolescents who had been treated as in-patients for school phobia and showed that over one third still had symptoms and were little improved. This poor outcome was likely if at the time of discharge from in-patient treatment the adolescent had not shown much response and if he had a particularly high IQ.

Thus it would appear that marked phobic fears in childhood can be a predictor of later adult phobic disorder, and that a history of school phobia in females can lead both to school phobia in any children they may have, and to an increased risk and earlier onset of agoraphobia in adult life. Good response to treatment for school refusal, particularly in the bright child, at the time of discharge from in-patient treatment is a predictor of better long-term outcome.

Once a phobic disorder is established in adulthood, it is important to know not only how well patients respond to specific treatments, but whether any improvement following treatment is maintained in future years. Early in the debate on the relative effect of behavioural therapy, as opposed to psychotherapy, it was suggested that response to behaviour therapy might be followed by symptom substitution, that is that new symptoms would appear because the underlying cause itself had not been treated, only the surface symptoms of that underlying cause. Therefore, in follow-up studies of behaviour therapy not only must immediate response to treatment be demonstrated, but also evidence of symptom substitution in the emergence of new symptoms not reported prior to therapy must be looked for. There are other questions that come to mind as well. In the long term, can cases which have been treated be shown to be significantly better in outcome than cases which have not been treated, where the condition has been allowed to follow its natural course? Do some phobias have a better long-term outcome after treatment than others?

In 1971, Marks reported a four-year prospective follow-up of sixty-five out-patients suffering from a phobic disorder for more than one year. Of this group, 55 per cent were suffering from agoraphobia, the rest from social phobias (22 per cent) and more specific phobias (23 per cent). The majority of the group were followed up for four years after they had stopped treatment. The results showed that most of the patients had obtained maximum improvement at the time of stopping treatment and did not change thereafter, and there was no evidence of symptom substitution. Irrespective of the type of phobia, 42 per cent of the group were showing significant improvement at the end of the study, and only 15 per cent had needed further treatment for depressive episodes, during which their phobic symptoms showed a temporary increase.

In 1979, Emmelkamp and Kuipers, from Groningen in Holland, followed up another group of seventy-five agoraphobics, again for four years. They found that improvement after behaviour therapy was maintained over the years, with some small gains. Of these patients, 75 per cent had improved two or more points on a five-point scale for their main phobia, and again there was no symptom substitution.

In 1980, Munby and Johnston from Oxford reported a follow-up study of between five and nine years on sixty-six patients suffering from agoraphobia. Three treatments were given: desensitization, flooding and psychotherapy, with home-based self-help programmes already described. They were able to contact 95 per cent of the original group. On most measures the patients were much better at follow-up than they had been before treatment began, and again most improvement occurred in the six months after treatment had stopped, with small further gains in a few patients. Once more, symptom substitution did not occur. They were able to show that this group had done well compared to untreated adult phobics, who, Agras had shown in 1972, improved little over five years. They also showed that those patients whose families were involved in the management programme and who organized this at home with self-help booklets did very well, because they had learned to become much more self-reliant, despite occasional relapses.

These outcome studies show that patients who are treated do better with treatment, and stay better, than people whose phobia is left to time alone. Improvement with treatment seems to occur mainly up to the time of stopping treatment and in the subsequent six months, although in a few cases there may be small improvements later. The type of phobia does not seem to affect the ultimate outcome, and symptom substitution does not occur with behaviour therapy, as predicted initially. Finally, the overall outcome for patients who are helped to understand the nature of their phobia and whose families are involved in self-help programmes initiated at home is very good, because such patients learn to cope better with occasional relapses.

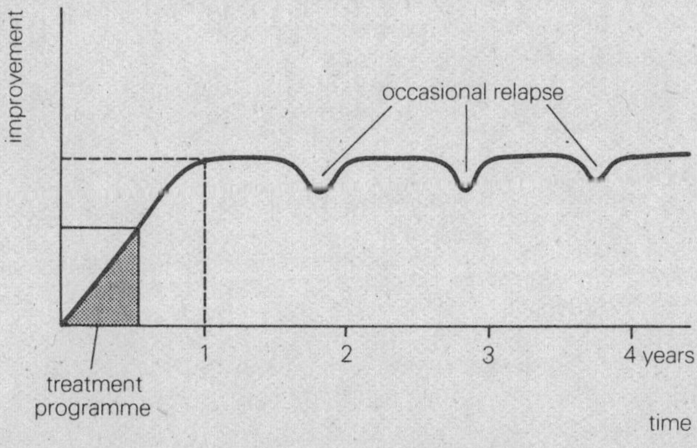

Fig. 10 Outcome over time

Overall, it would appear that various treatments are effective in phobic conditions and that improvement with such treatment is maintained. It is important that the patient and relatives should understand something of the nature of the disorder and its natural history, and should not rely too heavily upon professional support, but go on to develop a degree of self-reliance which comes from accepting a responsibility for the outcome of the disorder early on.

CHAPTER 9
A PHOBIA IN THE FAMILY

So far we have concentrated largely on the effect of a phobia on the individual sufferer, but any psychological and emotional disorder, perhaps even more than a physical disorder, must have an effect on other family members as well. Relatives respond with concern and sympathy to the initial outward effects of the phobia on the patient and try to give comfort and reassurance. Then, as the disability begins to make itself felt, they inevitably become involved in ways of helping the patient to get round their difficulties. They make allowances, go out of their way to be helpful and begin to take over tasks which the phobic cannot undertake. The phobic mother who cannot go shopping or easily leave the house will be helped by a husband, children or close friends who will do the shopping for her, and so on. In many ways this is very understandable – it is kind to the patient and the easiest way to keep family life going. Thus, the effect of the phobia on relatives and close family members is fairly obvious.

What is not so obvious is the effect of relatives and family members on the phobia. Without realizing it, the family can not only maintain the phobia once it is there, but can even initiate it in the first place. This may be difficult to accept and should be examined in more detail. The family can maintain the phobia by so arranging family life that the patient's avoidance behaviour is both accepted and legitimized – 'Mother can no longer do this for herself, so we will do it for her. It's not her fault; it's all due to the phobia.' By taking on these tasks for her, the family take away from her the pressing need to do anything about her phobia. As we have seen, anxiety, as well as upsetting us, is one of the strongest motivators to get things done. Taking away her anxiety also takes away her urge to deal with its cause. It is only later when the patient feels uncomfortable about her situation – 'Perhaps I ought to get something done about it; I can't really go on like this; I'm letting the others down' – or when relatives begin to feel it is time that the patient was better and able to take up her responsibilities again that the family doctor is asked to do something. However, by this time a compromise situation between the anxious patient and other family members has been reached, such that any treatment will inevitably mean discomfort and inconvenience both for the patient, who has to give up avoidance behaviour, and for relatives, who have to learn to stand back and let the patient slowly get into the swing of things again. To everyone's surprise, the family and patient may find themselves opting to go back to the more convenient compromise position, in which the phobic patient is not challenged any more and the phobia is reinforced. The family maintains the phobia.

Things are even more subtle than that. The family may call out the phobia in the patient and may in fact be largely responsible for it occurring in the first place. *Family theory* is concerned with the social interaction patterns within the family. The family is not a loose collection of independent individuals, but a closely organized system of interdependent ones. Each family member relies on, and is relied on in turn, by the others. Inheritance factors play their part and are handed down from one generation to the next. Within these genetic limits, emotional and psychological reactions build up over time so that each family becomes a unit for the education and acculturalization of its members. Families teach each other, consciously or unconsciously, what life is about, how problems should be dealt with and what happens when people cannot cope. There are in general terms healthy families in which the right helpful lessons are learned, but there are also sick families in which wrong unhelpful lessons are learned, or in which there is an excessive amount of physical or psychiatric illness handed on from one generation to another. It is possible therefore to speak of *phobic families* and *phobic marriages*. Just as an individual may have inherited patterns and for a variety of reasons become phobic, so a family unit or a marriage, for the same reasons, can become phobic. A phobic family is one in which there will be a large reservoir of inherited tendencies to be insecure and anxious, and to respond not by attacking problems, but by denying them or by running away from them; in other words, avoidance behaviour is seen as the best strategy for dealing with difficult problems and conflicts.

Within a family unit there is a subtle balance between needs and responses, between caring for and being cared for, between dealing with and failing to deal with problems. Certain family members take on specific roles as their contribution to family needs – the breadwinner, the home-maker, the decision-taker, parents who look after children, children who allow parents to look after them, and so on. The role of the mother remains central and vital. Her traditional task is to 'make the home' in the sense of holding things together while the father goes out to work. This traditional role is being challenged and altered, but even if the parents share the task between them, it is still common, because of the real differences in emotion and psychology in men and women, to see the mother as nurturant, that is, as the family feeder. Families can survive if the father leaves or is not there; it is less easy for families to survive if the mother leaves, or is incapacitated to a great degree. The redefinition of the feminine role in our society still has not gone far enough to alter the results of such family events significantly. Because of this central role, with all the expectations and pressures put upon her, it should not be altogether surprising that the mother most often carries the greatest emotional load, having to give more to the others than she perhaps gets back in return. Thus, within the family unit it is more often the mother who breaks down under the strain, with a psychological or an emotional disorder. This may be one explanation of why so many phobic patients, especially agoraphobics, are married females with young families. The phobic mother is demonstrating in her illness one aspect of the pressures which her family are trying to cope with.

There is also the concept of role-playing within the family. In a sense, a family, without realizing it, may elect one or other member to take on certain stresses and strains on behalf of the others, that is to take on an *illness role* in the family. This illness is not just the result of being under pressure, but acts as a distress signal indicating that all is not well and that something should be done to bring relief if something much worse is not to happen. Psychological disorders fit quite easily into this context. Thus, a phobic mother is not only showing the effects of strain upon herself, she may also be 'mirroring' strain in other members of the family. Just as in individuals the emergence of a phobia is in a sense a compromise solution to some continuing difficulty, so a phobia in a young mother may be a similar compromise solution to complex patterns of difficulty in the family, which cannot be expressed or revealed in any other way. This is not inevitable and true in every case, but it should be borne in mind when there is no other explanation, on an individual basis, why a particular person is phobic in terms of their own personal life history. In such circumstances the patient may be the 'spokesman' as it were of a phobic family.

It is in these senses that the structure of those families which can be called phobic families can both call out a phobia in a family member and also help to maintain it once the phobia has developed. The role of the phobic patient within such a family is a complex one. The patient's phobia is both signalling something about the family to others, that is serving family needs, but in itself becomes a potent source of frustration to those same family members. They begin by being sympathetic and understanding; they go on to make adjustments to the family life pattern; then, as the phobic symptoms continue in the patient, as undoubtedly they will until either the needs of the family are dealt with in some other way or the patient is sent for 'treatment', the family begins to get irritated and annoyed with the continuing state of disability in the patient. 'Why are you not getting better? Why hasn't the doctor done something for you? Why aren't you getting over it as your mother did?' and so on. The tragedy is that, as long as the phobia is serving needs in the family, we would not expect it to go away with time; we should expect the opposite – that the phobia will continue as long as the family helps to maintain it by encouraging avoidance behaviour in the patient, and as long as the phobia continues to serve undeclared and hidden needs in the family as a whole.

A family does not become phobic all of a sudden; this way of dealing with family problems and tensions evolves over time. It will begin in the very common phobic fears of childhood. These may be more marked than usual, or in some way cause more difficulty than in other families. Thereafter, one or other of the children may develop symptoms of school refusal, and the anxieties of parents and child become inextricably interwoven. As Berg showed, this school phobia may not resolve, but lead on to a full-blown phobic disorder in later adult life. Such a phobic family will now contain within it a larger representation of more than usually anxious and insecure members. Thus, anxiety and panic with avoidance behaviour will be experienced time and time again as the principal way of dealing with whatever problems may arise. All members of the family are exposed to this; a family culture of 'phobicness' is established by repetition and by expectation. Family members 'teach' each other to be potentially phobic. Which of them then develops the full-blown phobic illness depends on the variety of factors which determine the roles taken on within the family structure, but as the mother is in a centrally vulnerable position, she will often become the phobic patient within that family. Not all families with a phobic patient within them are phobic families. Individual cases arise for individual reasons, but as research into the family context of phobic illnesses continues, more is being understood of how these interacting relationship factors can play a major part in causing a particular phobia in a particular patient who comes for help.

In 1958, Eisenberg from Baltimore, in a study of twenty-six children suffering from school phobia, showed that these children were over-dependent on their parents, but that this over-dependence had been largely fostered by the parents themselves because of their own emotional needs. The mothers, in particular, he found to be more anxious than usual and to have had a poor relation with *their* mothers. These mothers had, as it were, been able to communicate to the children their own anxious attitude towards life. As well as cultural learning within these families, there could also be the influence of inherited anxiety proneness, an example of more than one factor operating at a time to produce a phobic outcome.

In 1976 Berg surveyed 786 women with agoraphobia, 299 of whom were married and had at least one child aged between seven and fifteen years. He showed that school phobia occurred to a greater extent in their children than would be expected (14 per cent in the age group eleven to fifteen years). Also, those agoraphobic mothers whose children developed school phobia had had the disorder themselves to an undue extent. A further finding was that a history of school phobia in these agoraphobic women was associated with an earlier onset of subsequent agoraphobia in adulthood, with more severe symptoms.

In 1979, Parker, in a follow-up of patients reviewed by Shaw in 1976 with phobic disorders and referred to the Oxford Psychological Treatment Research Unit, examined these phobic patients' perception of their parents' attitude to them. These patients perceived their parents as being both over-protective and uncaring. Those with social phobias saw both parents as over-protective and uncaring, while agoraphobics reported less maternal care. Intensity of social phobia was associated with greater maternal care and over-protection, whereas intensity of agoraphobia was associated with less maternal care and over-protection.

These reports show the *influence of parental characteristics* on the emergence of phobias in their children. Parental over-concern, reflecting an excessive anxious attitude on the part of the parents, especially the mothers, can lead to school refusal in adolescence and subsequent phobic disorders in later adult life. The over-protective attitude arose out of the emotional needs of the parents themselves; they were seen as ambivalent, that is blowing hot then cold, or else consistently uncaring in other respects. 'The fathers have eaten sour grapes, and the children's teeth are set on edge.'

In 1970, Agulnik made a study of the spouses of patients referred for phobic disorders to a Birmingham hospital. It had been found previously that there was generally a higher incidence of psychiatric disturbance than would be expected in the marital partners of patients with mental illness. This had been explained by saying that either psychiatrically disturbed people seek each other out or that the illness in one partner puts unreasonable strain on the other. In addition, over the years the impression had arisen that the spouses of psychiatrically ill patients had either not really understood the nature of the disorder, tending to react to it as if it was physical, caring for the symptoms in a protective way, or had appeared to be relatively detached from the patient's distress, with a fatalistic acceptance of the disorder. Did this happen with phobic disorders? Agulnik studied forty-eight partners of fifty married patients suffering from phobic disorders, largely agoraphobia. He found that the spouses of those phobic patients were not markedly neurotic on testing, and that any neurotic tendency in the spouse did not grow as the marriage continued. He believed that these findings, although not in accord with the previous general trends, nevertheless suggested that the phobic patient (the weak partner) had come to depend on the other (stronger) partner, who in turn was fortified by this dependence despite the limitations which it put on family life. Agoraphobic patients had been known to be extremely dependent, with a clinging characteristic – what Bowlby in another context has called 'anxious attachment'.

Hafner, in 1977, investigating the belief that the self-esteem and emotional well-being of one marital partner might depend on neurotic disability in the other, studied the effects of an intensive four-day behaviour therapy out-patient treatment programme on thirty-three married women with agoraphobia and on their husbands over a one-year follow-up. He concluded that he would not have learned about the husbands' difficulties and abnormalities without the lengthy and detailed follow-up procedure during which he was able to form a supportive and non-threatening relationship with the husbands, in the context of interviewing them ostensibly for the benefit of their wives. Denial of problems, and of disability and vulnerability, occurred very often, some husbands being unable to admit to difficulties even when these were clearly present.

Such *marital studies* in phobic disorders demonstrate that the influence and dependence of one married partner on the other can be vital in the origin and consequences of the phobia. Although one is clearly the patient with a psychiatric disorder, the other is often found to have their own internal difficulties, but these are denied and kept hidden. The apparently stronger partner can depend for his self-esteem and well-being on the manifest disability of the other. This is not so in all cases, but it should not be ignored as a possibility, not only because of the actual causation of the phobia, but also because of the importance of the marital partner in treatment programmes.

Several studies already mentioned have shown that treatment response and ultimate outcome are much better if the family is involved in a positive way with the treatment programme. This involvement reduces the potential isolation of the phobic person as the sick one of the family and recognizes the part which other family members may play in initiating and maintaining the phobia. The Oxford study of Munby and Johnston describes the involvement of the spouse in a *home-*

based treatment programme with explanatory booklets. Spouses can also be involved in *marital sessions* where the inquiry focuses on the effect of the phobia on the pair, and the effect of the pair on the phobia. It can be very hard for a husband to accept that he may be denying his wife an opportunity to escape from her phobia. New ways of relating to each other and new ways of sharing family tasks have to be spelt out in joint sessions, in which each can get across their feelings about the matter. Full *family therapy*, in which the key members of the nuclear family – the parents and their children who habitually live together under the same roof and share a corporate family life – are all involved in a treatment programme, can be necessary on occasion when the psychological organization of a phobic family continues to lock one or other member into the sick phobic role despite that person's attempts to escape from it. Such family sessions are difficult, but offer the possibility of discovering how each family member contributes to the problem and what each may have invested in keeping the phobic patient in the sick role.

Such an extreme position is relatively rare, and most treatments focus on the phobic patient. Individual sessions can be combined with occasional joint sessions with the spouse, to make sure that the couple are truly working in the same direction and that the spouse is giving the patient all the support and encouragement needed. A family diary is a useful way of exercising family involvement. The diary should set out clearly the agreed goals to be worked for, and should record progress towards these goals, emphasizing the gains rather than the failures. Scores can be given both for the degree of effort put into reaching the goals, and for the actual achievement. Occasional relapses and slip-backs are to be expected, and the forward momentum of the treatment programme must be sustained by the family.

We can summarize this in a set of *general family statements* which lay out a framework within which the individual patient will be treated:

(a) The patient must ultimately face the feared situation.
(b) The family must not take the easy way out which will isolate the patient and lead to avoidance.
(c) The family must support and encourage the patient to face fears.
(d) The family should help to monitor the patient's progress by the use of a family diary.
(e) The family must reward the patient for efforts made, to encourage further success.
(f) The family must help the patient to keep things in perspective, to avoid giving up prematurely.

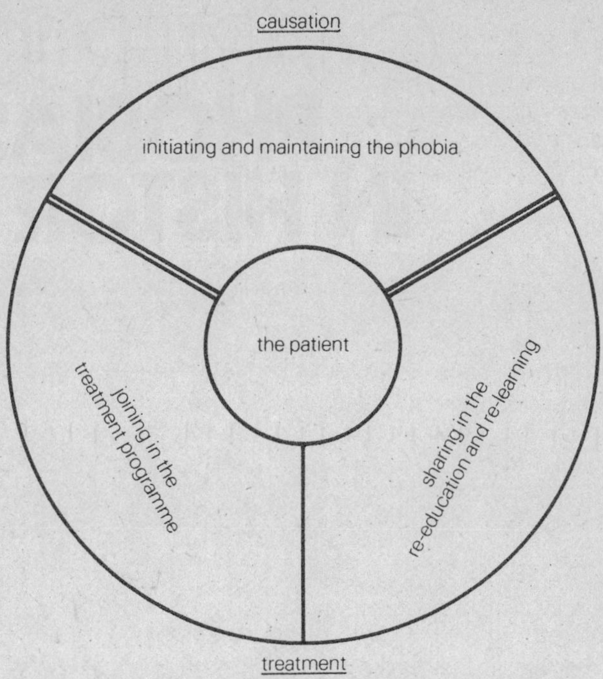

Fig. 11 The role of the family

We have now identified fully the ways in which the family is involved in the phobic disorder of one of its members. The particular family structure can play a part in both initiating and maintaining a phobic illness. Other family members must be involved in the programme of re-education (modification of attitudes) and re-learning (techniques of coping with the phobia), otherwise the patient becomes isolated in the sick role. Other family members, especially the spouse, should become involved in the treatment programme as co-therapists working with the patient, not only to provide encouragement and support, but also to take responsibility with the patient early on for the outcome of the disorder.

CHAPTER 10
PHOBIAS IN HISTORY

Although there is currently a great interest in phobias and they are more and more the cause of people coming for help, they are not recent events on the stage of history. References to conditions which, althougn not called 'phobic', are recognizable as such go back a long way in the human record. In medicine, as in so many other aspects of life, there are tides and fashions; certain conditions come to the surface and are exhaustively studied, occupying people's thinking to such an extent that they look like 'new illnesses'; it is forgotten that they have always been there, merged into the background of all the other disorders that affect people. Often, when a condition is becoming fashionable, it is given a catchy name which also creates the impression of something new. Thus it was with 'shell-shock', and now it is with 'agoraphobia' and 'housebound housewives'.

The origins of the terms 'phobia' and 'panic' go back into mythology: Phobos was an ancient Greek god who could strike terror into the hearts of his enemies, and Pan, the mischievous god of the woodlands, was attributed with the power to induce a state of uncontrolled behaviour in his devotees – a state of 'panic'.

The first reference to a phobia in a medical publication is thought to be the description of a clinical case by Hippocrates in the fifth century BC in his book *On Epidemics*. There is then a jump until the seventeenth century AD when in *The Anatomy of Melancholy* (1621) Robert Burton describes a man who dared not walk on his own from home for fear of fainting or dying, and another who could not cross a bridge, come near a pool of water or climb a hill lest he be tempted to hang himself, drown himself or throw himself off. Burton also comments that Octavius, who became the famous emperor Caesar Augustus, dared not sit alone in the dark, and records that Demosthenes, the famous Greek orator, suffered from great stage-fright. He was of the opinion that phobias were not under voluntary control – 'Take away the cause and otherwise counsel can do little good; you may as well bid him that is sick of an ague to be dry, or him that is wounded not to feel pain.' About the same time Shakespeare would appear to have been aware of phobias, for in *The Merchant of Venice* he speaks of 'some that are mad if they behold a cat'. Likewise, in 1650, René Descartes, the French philosopher, writes of 'the strange aversions of some who cannot endure the smell of roses, the sight of a cat'.

The next step forward was the publication in 1690 by John Locke, the English physician and philosopher, of his *Essay Concerning Human Understanding* in which he talks of the association of ideas and provides the first systematic description of a phobia and how it can come about: 'The ideas of goblins and spirits have really no more to do with darkness than light; yet let but a foolish maid inculcate these often into the mind of a child, and raise them there together, possibly he shall never be able to separate them again so long as he lives; but darkness shall ever afterwards bring with it those frightful ideas, and they should be so joined, that he can no more bear the one than the other.' Locke here anticipates much of the learning theory of phobias. In 1769, Le Camus, a French surgeon, in his book *Des Aversions* classified phobias according to the senses involved and quotes the case of James VI of Scotland and I of England, who was irrationally terrified of an unsheathed sword. This might be considered a case of learning in the womb, because on the night of 9 March 1566, some fifteen weeks before James's birth on 19 June, in the Palace of Holyrood, his mother Mary Queen of Scots, despite her pregnant state, was forced to watch as her favourite David Rizzio was stabbed to death before her eyes. Traumatic events cast their shadow before.

A more scientific approach to phobias began to emerge in the middle of the nineteenth century. In 1869, George Beard, an American psychiatrist, used the term 'neurasthenia' in the *Boston Medical and Surgical Journal* to describe a type of nervous exhaustion characterized by extreme loss of confidence and excessive fearfulness. This was followed a year later by the use of the term '*Platzschwindel*' by Benedikt to describe a particular dizziness that came on in public places. Karl Westphal then first used the term '*die Agoraphobie*' in 1872, and Raggi, in an Italian clinical review in 1877, used the term 'claustrophobia'. By the end of the nineteenth century there was a craze for classifying, according to classical nomenclature, a vast array of specific phobias with exotic names – taphophobia (fear of being buried alive), belonophobia (fear of needles), triskaidekaphobia (irrational fear of sitting down with thirteen people round a dinner table, popularly attributed to the fact that there were thirteen present at the Last Supper).

Sigmund Freud himself records that he had irrational fears to do with travelling; he was not only afraid of missing connections and would arrive ridiculously early for them, but irrationally terrified of what might happen if he did miss one. In 1895 he published a paper, *Obsessions and Phobias*, seeing a link between the irrationality of these conditions and the patient's awareness of how foolish the fears and obsessions were, though unable to resist them. Later in 1909 he published his paper 'Analysis of a Phobia in a Five-Year-Old Boy (Little Hans)'.

There are many anecdotal references to historic figures who over the years were known to have suffered from a phobia. Demosthenes, the orator, has already been mentioned; at the same time Damocles, the fourth-century Greek courtier of the sword fame, was said to be afraid of heights. Germanicus the general, and brother of the awkward Claudius, was afraid of cockerels. Henry III of France feared cats. The great John Bunyan writes in 1666 in his *Grace Abounding to the Chief of Sinners* of his delight in ringing the bells in Elstow church as a boy, but also of his guilt over this childhood pleasure which resulted in a phobic conviction that either a bell or the steeple itself would fall on him, as the tower of Ely Cathedral had fallen in the fourteenth century. There was a Russian general at the court of Catherine the Great who was afraid of mirrors and could not speak to his sovereign if there was one in the room. Manzoni, the Italian writer, was afraid to leave his home, and Feydeau, the French dramatist, was afraid of daylight. Samuel Johnson was preoccupied with a morbid fear of dying. Morel, the neuropsychiatrist, was afraid of heights. It is recorded that in 1794 a Mr Purrier craved to be excused from jury service because 'he comes very near fainting in crowded places'.

Phobias are not, therefore, new experiences, and all manners and customs of men have suffered from them. It is interesting that there is no historical reference to a woman having a phobia. This does not mean that they did not suffer from them, but probably reflects the sexist bias that only events happening to men are worthy to be recorded!

No doubt human beings have been phobic as long as they have been capable of being aware of themselves as vulnerable in the face of a potentially hostile and threatening world. All that has changed over the years is the balance between what is really dangerous to all and what is perceived to be so by a relatively few – the legion of the phobics.

Retrospect

Modern man's anxiety system, with its attendant fears and panics, arises out of our ancestral past, when to survive in a very hostile world it was vital to have an effective means which would alert us to danger and provide us with a method of immediate escape. Our anxiety system therefore is both an alarm and a means of mobilizing escape from danger. However, as life has developed and become more sophisticated the dangers to survival have become less obvious and less mechanistic. If we set aside the ever-present nuclear threat, most people feel threatened by others in terms of need for social success, social recognition and reward. The emphasis has shifted from a clear objective threat from without to a less precise subjective threat from within.

Phobias are an extreme example of this development; by definition the actual danger is minimal and the reactive anxiety response is inappropriate and irrational. The phobic person flees, not from any real danger, but from what he imagines to be the danger waiting for him. Thereafter, by avoidance he makes sure that he is not exposed to this imagined danger ever again.

The words 'imagined' and 'imaginary' are closely related to the idea of an image: a picture created in the mind. In order to think clearly and consciously we require building blocks of discrete thoughts which are best represented in images or pictures; if we can see something in our mind's eye we can feel clear about it; concepts which remain theoretical and cannot be pictured are difficult for most people. The more feelings can be expressed in pictures, the more powerful they become, with one exception – that feeling which is so powerful just because it is faceless, shapeless, half felt and half perceived in the dark – 'as I was going up the stair, I met a man who was not there; he was not there again today, I wish to God he'd go away.' The power of so many phobias lies in the fact that what is feared cannot be specified in images; it is a fear felt to be there, a fear of certain circumstances and consequences which cannot be spelt out and thus are doubly fearful because of this.

As creatures aware of our own consciousness we create images in the theatre of our own imaginations. At a fantasy level we project ourselves forward in time, anticipating what is going to happen to us. The imagery of these fantasies is powerful because it arises from archaic darkness inside each of us – the hobgoblins, ghosts and faceless terrors of childhood remain with us as adults but transformed into more sophisticated elements concerned with embarrassment, rejection, hurt, mutilation and the possibility of death. We must protect ourselves by taking avoiding action where we can, and learn by whatever means to banish these dark spirits from our imaginary world.

Because phobias are rooted in this theatre of fantasy, we must ultimately deal with those selfsame phobias there. Whatever means we use to eradicate the phobic tendency – drugs, psychotherapy, learning theory – there must at the end of the day be a change in the sufferers' attitude to themselves and to both the external and internal worlds. They must give up all thoughts of helplessness and of inevitability as far as the phobia is concerned and begin to see themselves as capable of some action, of some means of determining their own future. The fear cannot be charmed or wished away; it can only be faced. It must be confronted for what it is, acknowledged and dealt with. There is no other way.

The phobic person must not expect the phobic fear just to disappear, leaving them fearless. That is quite unjustified, and not what happens. The phobic person must learn to confront the fear and to survive despite it. It is the repeated survival in the face of the fear which slowly loosens its power over us. We cannot expect the fear to disappear, but we can expect to gain dominion over it, so that in the end it does not matter, because it does not limit our lives or predetermine our choices for us. The successful phobic is the person who can say: 'Yes, I was afraid and I ran away; now I am still afraid at times, but I can face my fear and it does not have power over me; as a result I feel so much better that I no longer fear my fear of my fear. It is slowly slipping away from me.'

The last enemy may still be death, but the greatest enemy of mankind along the road of life is the fear of fear itself.

Case histories

A school phobia *Malcolm, aged ten*

Malcolm was always a shy boy and did not play with the other children in his neighbourhood. He had some difficulty going to school in the first place, but eventually settled down to the school routine. Because he was quiet, he was picked on by the other children, and his mother would find him crying at home, but he would not say why. Malcolm's mother is herself a rather anxious woman who has tended to over-protect him and is clearly anxious every time he goes out of the house. She worries about him being knocked off his bicycle or getting into trouble with the other 'rough' children in the street. Malcolm began to complain of stomach aches, especially on Monday mornings, having been perfectly all right over the weekend. He began to refuse to have any breakfast and wanted to go back to bed when it was time to go to school.

His father usually takes him in the car on his way to business. Malcolm's mother tends to take his side, but his father says Malcom must face up to going to school like the other boys. At night Malcolm hears his parents quarrelling about this. Yesterday, things came to a head, with his father dragging Malcolm screaming out to the car, while his mother stood crying helplessly in the doorway, begging her husband not to force Malcolm to go to school. Malcolm's father is exasperated because he feels that Malcolm's mother is making everything doubly difficult and should be on his side in taking a firm stand with Malcolm. He is their only child, and clearly Malcolm's mother misses him when he is away at school. The teachers are aware of what is happening, and arrangements are being made for Malcolm to see the school doctor and the educational psychologist.

A separation anxiety *Mrs Anne Johnston, married, aged twenty-eight*

Mrs Johnston came to her doctor complaining of sleeplessness and general anxiety. This surprises her, for usually she feels confident and is rather a jolly, out-going person. However, in the last year or so, she has become more apprehensive and has been avoiding her friends and their invitations to visit them in their homes. She finds shopping a strain and encourages her husband to do it for her. While she is at home she feels better, but on reflection she feels very stupid and embarrassed by what is happening to her. She does not understand it, nor does her husband. Physically, she has not been very well, and they both wondered if this had something to do with it.

On closer questioning, it emerges that as soon as she leaves the house she begins to be apprehensive, and that the further she gets from home the worse it gets. If she immediately turns tail and runs for home she feels better, but very annoyed with herself. Now, even at home, she is beginning to be afraid of being left on her own. Her husband's business takes him away for periods at a time and she is dreading his next absence. It appears that being at home means feeling safe, and that home stands for the people who are closest to her emotionally – her mother, her father and her husband. She has nightmares in which she finds herself utterly alone, sometimes in the city, sometimes in the countryside. She cries out for help, but there is no one there. Being alone means that there is no one to protect her, no one to look after her if things go wrong. She has little confidence in herself and does not feel she could look after herself. She sees herself fainting or being ill, and there is no one there. The only safe place is home, home where there is always someone there to help her, or at least where in the past as a little girl there was always someone there to look after her. She is afraid of finding herself separated from the very people she needs for survival. She remembers being separated from her mother for a time when she was quite young because her mother was very ill.

A travel phobia *John Wilson, single, aged twenty-three*

John Wilson is an effective young teacher and likes to go abroad for his holidays. He wishes to go further afield and so is looking for package holidays with an air flight to Greece or North Africa. He rather embarrassedly confesses to his doctor of being terrified of aeroplanes. He has flown twice before and on both occasions ended up in a panic. He is frightened that it will happen again. He cannot look at pictures of aeroplanes, hear the sound of their engines or watch TV films of air flights without going into an acute panic – his heart thumps, his breathing is laboured, his hands sweat and shake, he feels like vomiting, and has to keep going to the toilet. This does not make any sense to him because he knows that, per passenger mile, flying is one of the safest means of long-distance travel; nothing has ever happened to him in an aeroplane or to anyone in his family or to anyone he knows. He realizes that his fear is quite irrational and is angry that it may stop him going abroad this year. Although aeroplanes are the worst, he is not happy about going in buses or trains, or in being in a car unless he is the driver. He has a fancy that the train or the bus will carry him off, away beyond his destination, but while he is driving the car he feels safer because he is in control of the vehicle.

Air flight is a nightmare because he has to sit surrounded by other people in a long thin metal tube that is hurled up into the sky, totally beyond his control. He has to sit back and abandon himself to the plane. He has fantasies of the pilot passing out or of a wing falling off, and sees himself plunging to his death. He wants to get rid of an excessive and irrational fear and to feel comfortable when he goes on holiday.

A specific phobia (fear of the wind) *Brian Kelly, married, aged twenty-six*

Brian Kelly is married with a young family. He is a successful business man. One night two years ago he woke up to find a gale had blown the slates off a neighbour's house and a tree had fallen across the street. He remembers at the time feeling a strange mixture of excitement and of apprehension. He thought no more about it, until he realized that he was anxiously watching the TV weather forecasts for signs of high winds in his locality. He worries that there might be a gale imminent and feels relief only when the current weather forecast rules this out. There have not been, in fact, any bad nights of high wind since, but he cannot stop himself worrying about the possibility. His wife tells him that he is silly because there is nothing really to worry about.

He is generally quiet and relaxed, but he does have a vicious temper if it is ever aroused. He finds it difficult to argue with people, especially with his wife, and prefers to take the easy way out, letting her have her own way most of the time. He knows that he does this, and he does not like to admit to it, but he cannot help himself. He likes things to be neat and tidy and worries at work when things seem to be getting out of hand and piling up. He likes to feel in control of his daily programme and resents any unwarranted interruptions.

It may be that his irrational fear of strong winds could represent a fear of his own internal anger; he certainly is afraid of what he might do if he were really to lose his temper with people, especially with his wife; he is frightened that he might hit out at her and knock her to the ground or cause her some damage. His doctor cannot help noticing that, on her medical file, his wife's name is given as 'Mary *Gayle* Kelly'!

A social phobia (a fear of eating out) *Mr Smithers, single, aged fifty-two*

Mr Smithers has worked all his life in a firm of accountants. He is a small, neat man who prides himself on his appearance and on the standard of his bookkeeping. Some people would call him a pedant because he is always on about 'things being done properly'. He has never married and lives a rather solitary life. He comes to his doctor because he feels what he calls 'depressed', but this turns out to be a dissatisfaction with life in general, and a specific problem in particular: he finds that he cannot go out to eat in public restaurants. He feels self-conscious and cannot relax, so much so that he feels sick even before he gets to the restaurant. He feels his face burning and is quite sure that everyone is looking at him. He feels awkward and knocks over the cruet or drops his cutlery onto the floor. His hands shake when he takes the menu, and he is sure the waiters notice this and are laughing at him.

While he is waiting for his order to come he does not know where to look; if he catches someone's eye, he feels dreadfully embarrassed. Panic begins to build up inside him and he has an irresistible urge to run from the restaurant. He did that once and created an awful scene: the tip of the table cloth caught in his jacket and he pulled everything onto the floor. He tries little tricks like humming nonchalantly to himself or reading a book, but he really cannot concentrate. When his meal comes he does not enjoy it and he cannot wait to get out of the restaurant. Waiting for his bill is purgatory for him. Having someone with him helps a little, but he is still afraid that he will make a fool of himself. If he takes a large whisky before he leaves home that helps too, but he is afraid of taking too much and then of appearing 'drunk' or of committing some social indiscretion.

An agoraphobia *Mrs Joyce Green, married, aged thirty-one*

Mrs Green is the first to admit that she has always been a bit nervous and anxious, but on the whole she has coped with life. She is married with three children and says that the marriage is a good one. There is only one problem: she cannot go to town to do the shopping. It began some two years ago. She remembers how it started. It was a hot, rather humid day and she found herself standing in the check-out queue at the local supermarket. There were friends coming to supper, and her trolley was rather fuller than usual. The queue seemed to be taking much longer; every shopper had a full trolley. She felt anxious, a little breathless, and thought she might even faint. She looked round desperately, but there was nothing she could do; she was caught in the queue and would not be able to escape until she had paid her bill. As she was hurriedly leaving the shopping area with her trolley, it caught the edge of a tall display of tinned goods and brought the whole thing tumbling to the ground. She fled in panic and in embarrassment.

She has never been back into that supermarket since, and nothing will make her. Now, whenever she thinks of the crowds in town and of the large department stores, she just cannot face the thought of going there. It is all too much for her. Her husband has to do all the shopping at the weekends or on late-opening nights, and he is beginning to feel annoyed with Joyce. He tells her she is being stupid, but she just will not go, even if he goes with her. She cannot face the thought of crowds of any kind. She has managed to go to the little corner shop nearby, but things cost more there than at the supermarket. She knows that it is unlikely that she really will faint, but she has an overwhelming sense of disaster if she goes into crowded places. She imagines herself doing something silly and drawing attention to herself. Everyone will gather round. Then she will not be able to breathe and will faint. She remembers that her mother's sister was like this and that she did not leave her house in ten years.

An illness phobia *Mrs Olive Grey, married, aged sixty-five*

Mrs Olive Grey has been haunted by a fear of illness all her life. She lost her father when she was quite young because of a heart attack, and she nursed her mother through her terminal illness with widespread cancer. Her husband, ten years her senior, is rather frail, but in reasonable health for his age. Mrs Grey frequently consults doctors with complaints of pain, discomfort, rashes, skin irritations, small swellings and so on. She is not suffering from ill-health, but is continuously afraid that she herself is going to have a cancer or some seriously incapacitating illness. Although her doctor tries to reassure her with frequent examinations and tests, she will be back again whenever some new symptom draws attention to the possibility of illness.

Mrs Grey, who is a genuinely religious person, is not afraid of death, although she will be sad not to be with her husband and her grown-up children and grandchildren; what she is afraid of is losing control of h dignity because of excessive pain or a disturbance of some bodil function. She remembers her mother soiling herself many times before she finally died. Mrs Grey sees illness as something that happens to people which, although not their fault, still carries some moral reproach. She feels that she should be fit and well in order to look after her husband and yet finds herself preoccupied with possible signs of something being wrong. It is the thought that she will not be able to cope with an illness that troubles her most, together with fear of pain and of disfigurement.

An animal phobia (fear of dogs) *Susan Campbell, single, aged eighteen*

Susan was a very apprehensive child; she was easily startled as a baby and could not be left alone in the dark. She suffered from frequent nightmares and grew up to be a timid, shy adolescent. Unlike other children she showed no interest in animals and would not look at pictures of animals in her books. She was terrified one day when her older brother put an earthworm down the collar of her dress, and since then she has not gone into the garden if there has been anyone else there to upset her.

She is now working as a typist in a local law office and quite enjoys her work. She gets on well with the other girls if they leave her alone. One thing makes her life a misery – the thought that she might meet a dog, any kind of dog, on her way to and from the office. Every morning her parents have to assure her that there is no dog in sight in the road, then walk with her to the bus stop. They have to wait until her bus comes and see her on to it. Susan arranges to be met by one of the other girls at the bus stop nearest to her place of work. If there is a dog in the street, they must cross over to the other side until the dog is out of sight. Once she gets to the office Susan goes into the toilet and counts up to ten, saying to herself 'There is no dog here; there is no dog here' before she can sit down at her desk and get on with her work.

She always brings a picnic lunch into work with her and eats it at her desk. She cannot go out to lunch with the other girls in case they meet a dog in the street. At first the others made fun of her, but now they have learned to leave her alone. She faces the same difficulties in reverse at the end of the working day and must be accompanied to the bus stop, to be met by her parents at the other end. The family have not been able to go away on holiday for five years now because of Susan's fear of dogs. In desperation, her father once gave her a puppy for her birthday, but Susan screamed hysterically until the puppy was taken away. She feels she will never lose her fear of dogs.

An obsessional phobia *Mrs Mary Brown, married, aged thirty-six*

When her children and her husband come home from school and from work, Mrs Brown insists that they take off all their outdoor clothes and have a bath. Afterwards they must put on clean clothes which have never been worn outside the house. All day she works hard at keeping the house spotless, and her kitchen shines because it is so clean. Before she uses any of the kitchen utensils, Mrs Brown has to wash them carefully and if possible boil them in a saucepan. Each pot and pan has to be scrubbed and washed in dilute disinfectant before she will use it. If something gets into the food while she is preparing it, she must throw it all out into the dustbin and start again. She knows that all this is unnecessary, but she cannot stop herself. She has been like this now for ten years, and there is no sign that she is getting any better. In the beginning her husband and children protested, but now they do what she asks, because they have learned from sad experience that this is the only way the family can stay together and survive.

Mrs Brown is not sure why she is doing all this; all she knows is that she must, if some tragedy is not to befall the family. She is not afraid of anything happening to her; she is haunted by the fear that because of some oversight on her part, some small omission, something terrible will happen to her family and it will be all her fault. She must constantly be on the lookout for potential danger from outside the house, before it can get in and do damage. She is wearing herself into the ground and knows it, but can do nothing to stop it. The only way she can get some relief is to go through all her procedures scrupulously, and even then there is always the doubt that she may have overlooked something. The family know that apart from this she is perfectly normal.

A pan-phobic reaction *Mrs Jean Grant, married, aged forty-five*

Mrs Grant is a frequent attender at her doctor. She has a large variety of complaints – coughs, colds, sneezes, headaches, constipation, poor appetite, insomnia and so on. Every so often she produces a new symptom to keep her doctor interested. She goes away each time reassured if her doctor listens to her and says that there is nothing seriously wrong to be concerned about.

Not unnaturally, she has always seen herself as an anxious, insecure, worrying person. She says jokingly that if she does not have something to worry about, then that worries her. Her family have given up trying to reassure her – they leave that to the doctor. Mrs Grant is shy and lacking in confidence; she does not like to go out into public places where there are a lot of people; someone might stop her to chat, and she would not know what to talk about. She always hangs back at parties and will avoid going if she can. She is easily upset by loud noises, bright lights and anything unexpected. Public transport terrifies her and she will not go into a lift or onto an escalator. She prefers to shop in the little local shops, and even here she will wait until the shop is empty before she will go in. She is afraid of animals and will not have a pet in the house.

She will not go to church with her husband, nor will she go to parent-teacher evenings at the children's school: she sends her husband in her place. He has the greatest difficulty getting his wife to go with him to his firm's annual Christmas dance, but once she is there she has been known to enjoy herself, though she will not admit it. She does not like to be left on her own at home after dark, and her married sister comes round to sit with her when her husband has to go out. Everything is a threat to Mrs Grant, and she will avoid all changes of routine if she can. She saw a programme once on television on agoraphobia; now she is afraid that she may have a phobia!

Glossary

Agoraphobia: an irrational fear of being in the open or in public places.
Anxiety: an unpleasant sensation of tension and uneasiness.
attached anxiety: anxiety consciously derived from some event or object
free-floating anxiety: anxiety not attached to any event or object
phobic anxiety: an irrational fear of some event or object
separation anxiety: fear from being separated from a safe base
signal anxiety: anticipatory anxiety, giving warning of threat
Behaviour therapy: a method of treatment based upon learning theory which modifies the patient's behaviour without concern for the deeper personal meaning of that behaviour.
Claustrophobia: an irrational fear of being in an enclosed space.
Depersonalization: an unpleasant sense of apprehension accompanied by a subjective feeling of being changed in oneself.
Desensitization: the use of relaxation to neutralize increasing strengths of anxiety-provoking stimuli; a type of behaviour therapy.
Ethology: the study of animal behaviour.
Fear: acute anxiety arising from imminent and perceived danger to oneself.
Flooding: placing the patient in the most anxiety-provoking situation and keeping them there until the anxiety response is exhausted; a type of behaviour therapy.
Learning theory: the understanding of behaviour as a series of associated or learned responses.
Modelling: going with the phobic patient into the real phobic situation and showing how to behave and how to cope with the anxiety.
Nervous: sensitive, easily disturbed, highly reactive, excitable.
Neurasthenia: nervous exhaustion leading to loss of confidence and to fearfulness.
Panic: acute fear, infectious fright, leading to hasty responses, including running about to no good purpose.
Pan-phobic reaction: a state of being irrationally afraid of everything in life; a state of severe loss of general self-confidence.
Phobia: an irrational fear of an event or object, which leads to avoidance of that event or object.

Phobic anxiety: anxiety which is irrational and inappropriate.
Phobic disorder: a true phobic illness with loss of function.
Phobic family: a family which habitually uses phobic defences as a way of dealing with inter-personal difficulties.
Phobic fear: common irrational fear, particularly in childhood.
Phobic marriage: a marriage in which both partners use phobic defences to deal with other problems.
Phobic reaction: a phobic experience as part of some other psychiatric illness or disorder, or a temporary reaction not going on to a true phobic disorder.
Psychoanalysis: the understanding of behaviour and experience in terms of personal meaning to the individual, arising from unconscious as well as conscious factors.
Psychodynamic: using psychoanalytic concepts in the understanding and treatment of behaviour disorders.
Psychotherapy: the use of a variety of psychodynamic techniques to bring understanding and relief to behaviour disorders.
Terror: extreme fear, which roots the person to the spot or leads to panic.

Further reading

The references in the text are taken mainly from the *British Journal of Psychiatry*.

On phobias

Muriel Frampton, *Overcoming Agoraphobia*, Thorsons, 1974.

Isaac Marks, *Fears and Phobias*, Heinemann, 1969.
Living with Fear, McGraw-Hill, 1978.

Charles Rycroft, *Anxiety and Neurosis*, Penguin Books, 1970.

Claire Weekes, *Self-Help for Your Nerves*, Angus and Robertson, 1962.
Peace from Nervous Suffering, Angus and Robertson, 1972.
Agoraphobia, Angus and Robertson, 1977.

Of general interest

Michael Argyle, *The Psychology of Interpersonal Behaviour*, Penguin Books, 1968.

Eric Berne, *Games People Play: The Psychology of Human Relationships*, Penguin Books, 1968.

Anthony Storr, *The Integrity of the Personality*, Penguin Books, 1970.
Human Aggression, Penguin Books, 1971.

Further information and literature on phobias can be obtained from: The Information Officer, MIND (National Association for Mental Health), 22 Harley Street, London W1N 2ED (tel. 01-637-0741).

Some useful addresses

The Centre for Behavioural Psychotherapy, 22 Queen Anne Street, London W1

The Open Door Association, c/o 447 Pensby Road, Heswall, Merseyside LI6 9PQ (tel. 051-648-2022).

The Phobics Society, 4 Cheltenham Road, Chorlton-cum-Hardy, Manchester M21 1QN (tel. 061-881-1937).

The Phobic Trust, c/o 25a The Grove, Coulsdon, Surrey CR3 2BH (tel. 01-660-0332).

Mr Tony Elliot, 1 Oban Road, Chilwell, Nottingham (stamped addressed envelope).

MIND (National Association for Mental Health), 22 Harley Street, London W1N 2ED (tel. 01-637-0741).

Index

More about Penguins and Pelicans

Also by Ross Mitchell

DEPRESSION

Depression is one of the most common contemporary problems. But what exactly do we mean by the term? In this invaluable book Ross Mitchell looks at depression as a mood, as an experience, as an attitude to life and as an illness. He examines the organic, psychological and social roots of depression, laying particular emphasis on the early relationship between mother and child. His argument is illustrated by a number of case histories, and an important concluding chapter focuses on the role of both volunteer and professional in caring for the depressed.

A selection of books on Psychology and Psychiatry

THE FOUR FUNDAMENTAL CONCEPTS OF PSYCHO-ANALYSIS

Jacques Lacan

Jacques Lacan's writings have provoked intense controversy in French psychoanalytic circles, requiring as they do a radical reappraisal of the legacy bequeathed by Freud. In this volume, based on addresses to a larger and less specialized audience than ever before, he wanted to discuss 'the major concepts on which psychoanalysis is based', namely: *the unconscious, repetition, the transference* and *the drive.*

THE MYTH OF THE HYPERACTIVE CHILD
And other Means of Child Control

Peter Schrag and Diane Divoky

'A well-researched and thoughtfully argued brief intended to stimulate action against the widespread use of drugs, psychological testing, and behaviour modification used by agents of the state to control children's lives and undermine their rights' – *The New York Times Book Review*

THE LANGUAGE OF MADNESS

David Cooper

The language of madness, maintains David Cooper, expresses both a need, and a challenge to the world which fails to recognize that need. It therefore demonstrates our corporate failure to bring together our sexuality, our lives and our autonomy. Cooper claims that we must accept this indictment and points to ways in which we can rectify the situation.

Psychology in Pelicans

THE PSYCHOLOGY OF HUMAN AGEING

D. B. Bromley

Infant and adolescent psychology have been very thoroughly explored, but the study of ageing lags behind. This new introduction to human ageing and its mental effects is written by the Scientific Advisor in Gerontology to the Medical Research Council, and is of importance to both the student of psychology and the layman.

THE PSYCHOLOGY OF LEARNING

R. Borger and A. E. M. Seaborne

Only a small part of learning takes place in schools. In this book two psychologists discuss the laws which seem to govern the process of learning in its widest sense. They also provide a thorough survey of programmed learning techniques and the newer developments in the formal teaching of schools and universities.

THE PSYCHOLOGY OF STUDY

C. A. Mace

An explanation of the mental processes by which we all 'read, mark, learn and inwardly digest' information of all kinds. There are chapters on perception, memory, original thinking, concentration and preparation for exams.

THE PSYCHOLOGY OF THINKING

R. Thomson

The achievements and limitations of recent studies into 'thinking' are discussed and evaluated. The direct experimental investigation of adult thought processes, and the intelligent behaviour of animals, are also dealt with.

More books on Psychology and Psychiatry

FREUD AND HIS FOLLOWERS

Paul Roazen

'An extremely rich book . . . It would seem to be essential reading for all who are interested in the history of psychoanalysis or the history of ideas in the twentieth century' – *Guardian*

Paul Roazen interviewed more than seventy people who had known Freud and probed minutely into Freud's home-life, his friends and disciples – Jung, Ernst Jones, Ruth Mack Brunswick, Melanie Klein among others – to reveal the rich, productive world where 'the theories that were to revolutionize what we think of ourselves' took root and ripened.

THE PIGGLE
An Account of the Psychoanalytic Treatment of a Little Girl

D. W. Winnicott

From the age of two until the age of five, the Piggle – seriously disturbed by the birth of a younger sister – visited the late Dr Winnicott on sixteen occasions. A verbatim account of her visits is accompanied by illuminating excerpts from letters written to the analyst by the child's parents and an invaluable commentary by Dr Winnicott.

MUSEUMS OF MADNESS
The Social Organization of Insanity in Nineteenth-century England

Andrew T. Scull

Andrew Scull traces the developments in the treatment of insanity in nineteenth-century England, from the iron cages of Bethlem to the non-restraint policies of the reformers. He follows the progress of the movement for reform, analyses the motives of its opponents, assesses its impact on the 'mad' trade and asks what proof have we that the shift from 'madness' to 'mental illness' has been accompanied by any progress in the treatment of the insane.

Also published by Penguins

HUMAN AGGRESSION

Anthony Storr

In this monograph the author of *Sexual Deviation* and *The Integrity of the Personality* writes both as a psychotherapist and as a human being living in an age when 'The End is Nigh' could well be the truth. But the coin of aggression, as he shows, bears two faces. As a positive and natural drive he discusses its normal role in the social structure of both animals and men and its function in childhood, adult life, and sexual relations: in its negative aspect he considers hostility in relation to depressive, schizoid, paranoid, and psychopathic personalities.

HOW CHILDREN FAIL

John Holt

'It is possibly the most penetrating, and probably the most eloquent book on education to be published in recent years. To anyone who deals with children and cares about children, it cannot be too highly recommended' – *New York Times*

'John Holt has done a good and necessary job. A very good book indeed' – A. S. Neill

SUCCESS AND FAILURE IN LEARNING TO READ

Ronald Morris

No educational issue has given rise to such a mountain of research and argument as the teaching of reading. The debates, the texts, the hypotheses continue to appear, and unlike many complex educational issues they very largely appear in public. For reading is perhaps the major ground on which the public at large chooses to question and challenge the teaching profession. Is Johnny reading or not? And if not, why not?

More books on Psychology and Psychiatry

THE DIVIDED SELF

R. D. Laing

'It is a study that makes all others I have read on schizophrenia seem fragmentary . . . the author brings through his vision and perception, that particular touch of genius which causes one to say "Yes, I have always thought that, why have I never thought of it before?"' – *Journal of Analytical Psychology*

NEW HORIZONS IN PSYCHOLOGY, VOLUME ONE

Ed. Brian M. Foss

Genetics, motivation, drugs, operant conditioning, programmed learning and behaviour therapy are some of the new developments in psychology affecting scientific thinking and influencing our lives today. This expert volume is both a progress report and an indication of future directions.

THE SAVAGE GOD
A Study of Suicide

A. Alvarez

This controversial study of this often taboo area of human behaviour embraces both cultural attitudes and the development of theoretical studies, giving a broad basis for Alvarez's examination of suicide from the perspective of literature. Here, he follows the black thread leading from Dante through Donne and the Romantic Agony, to Dada and the Savage God at the heart of modern literature.